MANIC MAN

MANIC MAN

How to Live Successfully with a Severe Mental Illness

Jason Wegner

and

Dr Kerry Bernes

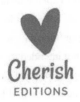

Cherish
EDITIONS

First published in Great Britain 2021 by Cherish Editions

Cherish Editions is a trading style of Shaw Callaghan Ltd & Shaw Callaghan 23 USA, INC.

The Foundation Centre

Navigation House, 48 Millgate, Newark

Nottinghamshire NG24 4TS UK

www.triggerhub.org

Text Copyright © 2021 Jason Wegner

British Library Cataloguing in Publication Data

A CIP catalogue record for this book is available upon request from the British Library

ISBN: 978-1-913615-41-3

This book is also available in the following eBook formats:

ePUB: 978-1-913615-42-0

Jason Wegner has asserted his right under the Copyright, Design and Patents Act 1988 to be identified as the author of this work

Cover design by BookCollective

Typeset by Lapiz Digital Services

For those who live with a mental illness:
It can get better.

FOREWORD

To Jason, "life-storming" was how he described the 55 minutes of non-stop, faster-than-I've-ever-heard-anyone-speak, completely incoherent ramblings contained in our first meeting. To me, bipolar I disorder was the diagnosis and at that moment, Jason was clearly in a heightened manic state. With the support of his parents, he was hospitalized shortly thereafter.

Jason was actually dragged in to see me by his very worried parents—he genuinely thought he was coming to "shrink the shrink". This highlights a common theme and some of the most significant barriers in treating severe mental illness: recognition of the illness by the family (to seek diagnosis and support), acknowledgment of the illness by the patient (to seek stabilization and treatment), and compliance with the treatment plan and goals. Without a strong medical team, family support, access to mental health resources, appropriately prescribed pharmaceuticals, psychotherapy and eventual compliance, these patients frequently experience lives filled with addiction, unrealized education and career goals, relationship failures, and poverty. Sadly, homelessness is not uncommon. After experiencing 18 months of hard work and many ups and downs, Jason truly beat the odds stacked against him, which led me to suggest his story needed to be told. For anyone living with, or who loves someone they suspect is suffering from a severe mental illness, this book is a must read.

I have been a board-certified clinical psychologist for nearly 20 years and have seen untreated – and poorly treated – bipolar disorder exert a heavy toll on patients and their families. Happily, Jason's story is one with a positive outcome. From a very ill 20-year-old whose diagnosis was met with distrust, paranoia, denial and anger to an extremely accomplished 24-year-old who is stable, happy, healthy and a straight-A student at university, this book will give you, as the reader, insight into a world that few know about and fewer understand. You will have the opportunity to enter Jason's world and bear witness to the progression of Jason's descent into mental illness, diagnosis, treatment, and how he turned it into post-traumatic growth. Jason genuinely demonstrates how all of us can not only overcome the hardest challenges in life, but become stronger in the process.

Dr. Kerry Bernes
B.Ed., M.Sc., Ph.D., R.Psych., ABPP
Board Certified in Clinical Psychology
(American Board of Professional Psychology)
Professor
Faculty of Education
University of Lethbridge

CONTENTS

PROLOGUE

I walked into the bathroom and accidentally saw my reflection in the mirror, which instantly freaked me out.

"Dad, Dad, are my eyes okay? Are my eyes okay?"

"Yes, of course. There's nothing wrong with them."

"Are they super dilated?"

"No, Jason. They look fine."

I couldn't fall asleep, so, naturally, I grabbed five books off my bookshelf and went outside to the backyard to do some night reading. "Might as well put this insomnia to good use!" I said to myself. I cracked open *The Way of the Peaceful Warrior* by Dan Millman, and began trying to read under the night sky, using my phone as a reading light. A few moments later, two paramedics entered my backyard. They asked me how I was doing and why I had writing all over my arms, legs and shorts. I said, "I'm doing just fine, and the writing is for the Vow of Silence campaign. Who the hell are you guys?"

"We're from the hospital and wanted to check on you."

"I've never felt better in my life," I replied.

I saw my mother in her white robe standing on the deck, watching the scene unfold. The paramedics asked me to come with them, and I was completely compliant. I acted extremely politely and as normal as possible, so they wouldn't take me away. They told my mother there was nothing they could do as I was not displaying any behaviour that would suggest I was a harm to myself or others. My mother continued to plead with them to take me away, citing my erratic behaviour over the last few weeks. I got frustrated with the discussion about my well-being and decided to light a cigarette, knowing it would agitate my mother. Exasperated, my mother challenged me, "If you're feeling so 'spectacular', then prove you're okay by seeing a doctor tonight."

Always up for a challenge, I accepted her plea, because I knew, beyond a doubt, there was nothing wrong with me. In fact, I believed I had tapped into supernatural powers of human potential. I had never felt so good and so efficient in my entire life. However, I had many things to do at 2:30am on a Sunday evening in August, so I began negotiating with the paramedics about not going to the hospital. After much deliberation, they agreed to let me out of the ambulance once we got to the hospital; they said they would let me take a cab ride home immediately. I soon found out this was a lie.

At the emergency room, I was agitated at not being allowed to leave, and began pleading my case to the younger paramedic, who seemed more sympathetic to me. I'll never forget thinking that he was a messenger from the future who had time-travelled back to 2017 to comfort me in my moment of distress. He said, "You're just ahead of your time, son." Considering that he was warning me of this from the future naturally made me feel ultimately defeated. The older paramedic then guided me to my "cell" for the night – a fluorescent-lit, grey concrete room, with a solitary bed in the middle and a surveillance camera in the top left corner.

To prove my sanity and talents, I began performing Pink Floyd's *The Wall* into the blinking red light of the surveillance camera. They hadn't confiscated my iPod, so I sneakily put the album on and listened to it with my hood up to hide it. Singing my heart out and acting the scenes of the rock opera to my audience, I completed the whole first half of the album before I took off my hood and screamed to the camera, "See, you fools! You thought I was performing that album verbatim, but I had my iPod the whole time! I am the world's greatest actor and greatest spy!" The medical staff promptly entered the room and confiscated my iPod, which I should have expected; I was getting very tired and didn't feel like fighting.

However, my lethargy disappeared immediately when a doctor entered the room with two blue pills, which he shoved in my face. I obviously refused this attempt at pumping me full of mind-controlling drugs. I did not want to sacrifice my super-powered intelligence in any way. I refused the drugs until he left me alone, and I demanded my release from the prison, but to no avail. I was being held against my will and felt utterly helpless. They wouldn't let me have *my* medicine either, because marijuana was not deemed appropriate for my state of being. Distraught, I finally drifted off to sleep.

The next morning, I was wheeled into the acute psychiatry ward of the hospital, where I was diagnosed with a severe mental illness: bipolar I disorder, and was subsequently insitutionalized for 57 days.

Bipolar I disorder is a mental illness that causes unusual shifts in mood, energy, activity levels, concentration and the ability to carry out day-to-day tasks. These moods range from extremely elevated and "up" – known as manic episodes – to very sad and "down" – known as depressive episodes. Specifically, there are two major types of bipolar disorder, bipolar I and bipolar II. Bipolar I is defined as having a severe manic episode with symptoms that include rapid thinking, pressured speech, insomnia, increased energy, grandiose ideas, excessive spending and substance abuse. Bipolar II is defined as a pattern of depressive and hypomanic symptoms without a full-blown manic episode. Bipolar II is not typically treated with hospitalization, while bipolar I usually requires hospitalization.

Writing this book was part of my treatment – diving deep into the story of how I ended up in hospital, and confronting my actions and behaviours during my manic episode, has allowed me to come to terms with my severe mental illness. Such extreme exposure therapy has resulted in me experiencing post-traumatic growth and having a better life than before my diagnosis of bipolar I disorder.

PART I

HYPOMANIA

1

GROWING UP

Growing up in Alberta, Canada, I had a normal childhood. I played ice hockey and baseball, did well in school and had good friends. By the time I was 15, I had become obsessed with ice hockey. I wanted to play in the NHL (National Hockey League) one day, so I quit baseball and began training with Trevor Hardy at HARD Training. There, my commitment to growing as a player was supported by a training staff that included Jordie Deagle and Justin Kanigan. They both pushed me that first summer at HARD Training – harder than I had ever been pushed.

I also developed a love of reading while I was there. Jordie was studying Political Science at Carleton University in Ontario, and went on to become Canadian Prime Minister Justin Trudeau's communications advisor. Jordie convinced me to start reading books by telling me, "It will help you pick up chicks." Naturally, I began reading a lot.

This new-found love of reading eventually influenced my professional career, as I went on to study to become an English language arts teacher in university. That summer of being 15 was also when I was introduced to one of my heroes, the American author, coach, speaker and philanthropist, Tony Robbins.

My HARD Training coach, Trevor is by no means tech-savvy, so that summer he had me put some music and audiobooks on his iPhone. One of the audiobooks he asked me to add was by Tony Robbins. Trevor told me that Tony's stuff would be right up my alley, so one day, when I was in a bookstore and saw Tony's giant face staring at me from the cover of *Awaken the Giant Within*, I picked up a copy. Now, hockey players are not a dumb breed by any means, but sometimes the stereotype that they only think about the game and picking up chicks rings true. So, when I was 15 and playing Bantam AAA hockey, and reading books at the front of the bus on road trips, I definitely got teased by the other players and the coaches. It was just "irregular" behaviour. I never cared much about being ostracized for wanting to grow as a person though, so I always shut the teasing out and laughed along.

With Tony Robbins' material, I became obsessed with personal growth. I wanted to make the NHL, and I thought that having a mental edge would be the key. Tony has an exercise in his *Get The Edge* programme called the "Hour of Power". While walking you begin chanting positive phrases to ingrain them in your mind. For example, he'll have you shout, "I AM GREAT IN EVERY WAY" and "ALL I NEED IS WITHIN ME NOW!" Buying into the concept for a few weeks, I would get up at 5am before school and walk around the neighbourhood, shouting "I AM THE CHAMPION! ALL I NEED IS WITHIN ME NOW!" It was exhilarating, and definitely got me out of my comfort zone. I eventually gave up the Hour of Power walks because, although I was reeling from the experience, they did make me tired for school.

I had my most successful hockey season when I was 16 and playing for the Midget AA Hounds. The coach I had that season was the best I would ever have. He really had an attention for detail, and embedded a winning culture in our locker room. We had a great team that year and went all the way – winning the league and provincial championships. In our season ending exit meeting, the coach said one of the most inspiring things anyone has ever said to me: "Jason, I was telling another player that no matter what you do, whether it's becoming a businessman or a gravedigger, you will be the best damn gravedigger around." The coach saying I would be the best at something gave me so much confidence as a young person that I have never forgotten that day.

I trained harder than ever that summer because I wanted to make the Midget AAA team the following fall, as that league springboards a lot of players into junior hockey, which is the next step toward the NHL. However, the coach who had complimented me ultimately went with a younger player and cut me from the team. I was beyond devastated. It felt like my hockey career was over. I cried pretty hard that night, until I called Trevor. He set me straight, saying that I could have an even better opportunity with the Midget AAs – getting more ice time and becoming a leader on the team. This instantly changed my mindset, and that same night, I drove across town to meet my new coaches with the Midget AAs. I told them I was all in and wanted to take the team to the championship again. They were so impressed, I even became team captain.

However, my expectations and goals were not well met. Our talent level and the experience of the coaching staff did not match my high aims for the team. I began clashing with other players and the coaching staff because I wanted to win so badly. I wanted the practices and the games to be as professional and intense as the previous season's, but they weren't. It didn't take long for the team to turn on me, as I was too intense for many of them. Most of the players and the coaching staff just wanted to have fun and didn't obsess about winning as much as I did.

Before a game in November, only two months after the season had started, the coaches called me into their office and took my captaincy away. I was very embarrassed, but I played the game anyway. It was a low point in my life because I thought I was a good leader – but good leaders know how to work with their team, and I had become a very negative captain. I didn't have much fun that season, and I was disappointed when I didn't get called up to the AAA team after one of their players broke their leg. I thought that would be my opportunity to move up, but I had suffered a concussion from a dirty hit at the same time as the other player had broken his leg. The AAA team decided to play one player short for the rest of the season, and, aside from a few call-ups, I never got an opportunity to play for them full-time.

I gradually began to re-evaluate my hockey career. Playing junior hockey looked unlikely because I wasn't getting scouted by any teams and I wasn't having fun with the game anymore. I took it too seriously, to the point that I was getting frustrated all the time. Before my 18th birthday in January 2015, I decided that I would shift gears from trying to be an NHL player to trying to find a different career. I also decided that I wouldn't take hockey so seriously anymore and would just play for fun. This turned out to be the best thing I could have done, and with my attitude change the game became enjoyable again. At the end of the season, my head coach was so proud of the way I had changed my attitude that he gave me my captaincy back for the last game. I was really proud in that moment too, as I felt that I had grown as a person throughout that season.

Being 18 and not so focussed on hockey, I decided to get a good job during my last semester of high school. My dad was friends with a local bar owner in town, and in February 2015, I began working as a bouncer at a sports bar. I loved that job. There were sports on all the time, concerts playing and, of course, women everywhere, especially on the staff. I was still in high school, but I felt way more mature than my fellow students. I was working in one of the top bars in the city, making $20 an hour to start. I felt like a king, and I would eventually meet my queen a few shifts into the job.

2

THE GIRL

At first, I hadn't taken much notice of the beautiful blonde waitress with the British accent. I thought she was gorgeous, but I assumed she had a boyfriend. I was also attracted to a few other waitresses, but I was still in high school, so I didn't think I had much of a chance with any of them. But, one night as we were closing up, a waitress friend pulled me aside and asked if I had a crush on any of the other waitresses. Not wanting to give myself away, I didn't say, "Well, all of them!" I played it cool and said, "I don't know, why does someone like me?"

The waitress continued to be coy and said, "I don't know, maybe," with a big smile on her face. Originally, I thought she was talking about herself, so I guessed her, and she laughed and said no. She was 23 and knew I was 18, so I didn't have a chance. I eventually guessed, "The Brit with the blonde hair," and I was right. I couldn't believe it. Her name was Layla, and she was one of the nicest, most gorgeous girls I had ever met, and she had a crush on me! I invited her for a drink after work on St Patrick's Day, and she excitedly agreed.

We instantly hit it off that night. I had already decided I wanted to study to be an English teacher, because I was so inspired by my Grade 11 and 12 English teacher, Greg. He had been teaching at the same high school for 42 straight years! He was an absolute pro and instilled a love for the subject in me that I have to this day. I credit my career choice to Greg a lot, as he always seemed so happy in his job. Layla had also chosen to teach, and was doing her teacher training when we met. She was 22 — I was 18, and I did not want her to find out how young I was.

St Patrick's Day was on a Tuesday, so I had school the next day at 8am. We talked until the bar closed at 3am and luckily my cover was not blown. I was going away that weekend for a hockey tournament, but we agreed to meet again when I got back. I was pumped, and my confidence was at a level ten. Here I was in high school, and I had a date with a university student — I did not want to mess it up.

We texted back and forth all weekend, and I didn't give away that I was playing minor hockey. I think Layla thought I was a junior hockey player or something. When I came home on Sunday, she agreed to have dinner with me, and I was to pick up her up at her westside home. I frantically cleaned my GMC Jimmy, so I'd have a clean car to pick her up in. I remember my dad saying, "You must really want to impress this girl!"

I took her to a nice restaurant and foolishly ordered the cheeseburger. It was a messy meal, but I tried to eat as neatly as possible. I don't think she noticed, but I was very nervous. And the burger had an onion on it, so I was really self-conscious of my breath. After the meal, she left for the restroom, and I desperately asked the waitress for a breath mint or a piece of gum; she didn't have any. I was very embarrassed, but Layla didn't notice anything. To this day, I always have mints on hand.

I drove her back home and said goodnight, not making a move or anything because of the onion breath I thought I had. She asked me, "Can I kiss you?"

I said, "Yeah, of course!" and we had our first kiss. We dated for eight months, and she was the first girl I said "I love you" to.

Going into my first year of university (and Layla's last year of university), I learned a lot about how to be a good student. I credit Layla for much of my success as a student because, instead of acting like a first-year, I acted like a fifth-year. I hung out with her friends, studied lots and learned terrific study habits. In my first semester of university, I achieved an A, three A-s and one C+. The C+ was for a geography class that I had no interest in, but I was proud of the other four classes. Layla and I had a terrific relationship, but it was destined to end – our worldviews were too different. I was a young first-year student, and she was a more mature, graduating student. It all came to an end when she had to decide where she wanted to go for her last placement as a student teacher. She was from a small town away from the city and had already done a placement in the city. I didn't want to hold her back, so I encouraged her to make the choice that would give her the best chance at a successful career. She chose to do her placement close to her hometown so she could live with her parents and focus on the work.

I will never forget the night we broke up. I live on the north side of town, and to get to the west side you have to go down the only connecting bridge to the west side of the city. We had agreed to meet at her place to "have a talk", and I knew she was going to break up with me. When I was about to go down the bridge towards her place, a cop car raced in front of me and blocked the access to the bridge because of an accident. I had to wait over an hour in a parking lot waiting for the bridge to open. I knew I was destined to get my heart broken. Finally, the bridge opened, and I was able to get to her place before my shift at the sports bar. Our "talk" was short and painful. She said the timing sucked – because we were both at two different stages of life it wasn't going to work out. I took my things and had an emotional walk back to my car. I cried on the way to work, but wiped my tears before entering the bar. I bottled it all up and repressed my feelings.

Recently promoted, I was on a bartending shift that night. I really liked bartending, as it was more interaction with people and even better money than working as a bouncer. On this night, I definitely didn't feel like talking. But I did tell my friend and regular at the bar, James, what had happened. James was a great guy who had a lot of experience with women and the bar industry. He would later work for the bar and take me under his wing as a young bartender. On this night, his advice was simple: "Forget about that girl and live it up, Jason. You're a young guy who just started university, and you're a bartender! The world is at your feet, kid." I guess it made me feel a little better, but I had just lost the girl of my dreams, and I didn't feel like talking about other girls. But I got through the shift that night and tried to pick myself up the next day, trying to focus on the freedom of being a single man again.

Party Time

Those first few months after the break-up were really hard. Everything I had that reminded me of Layla – postcards, notes, pictures – I put in a box and had my mom stash it away somewhere. I also deleted everything on my Facebook page that left a trace of her. I would learn later that repression and avoiding triggers is the worst thing I could have done, but I didn't know any better. For almost three years, every time I heard a song by Michael Jackson or Bon Jovi, artists we had regularly listened to together, I would immediately change the station. I almost had a breakdown one day in class when a song by one of them came on during a video. It was not healthy. And because I didn't get over the break-up, I didn't look for any other meaningful relationships; I only had flings. There are a handful of awesome girls I could have potentially dated had I not still been hung up on my ex. But, like many people, I sought to repress those feelings with drugs and alcohol.

Being a bartender at a top bar in the city, I was making good money and was in a highly social environment. On nights off, I would hit the bar scene, looking to pick up girls for one-nighters and drink with friends to have a good time. I spent a lot of money on booze, but I was making so much that I didn't really care. I was saving money for other things, but my disposable income was still high. In hindsight, I should have saved more, but I was 19 – just a kid. I was obsessed with the lifestyle of a bartender. I felt like Tom Cruise out of the movie *Cocktail*, and was on top of the world. However, deep down I was still sad about losing Layla. But I repressed those feelings deep down so I wouldn't have to worry about them.

3

TEACHER ADVERSITY

School was still going well when I turned 19. I had such good study habits and so much energy that I was able to get excellent grades taking five classes and working three six- to eight-hour shifts at the bar. I was fairly sure I wanted to be a teacher at this point, but I wanted to *make* sure. I didn't want to waste a year of school taking English classes when I could be working towards a business degree, which was another interest of mine. So, I decided to take the first education class available that summer, which was Education 1000. The class was an introduction to teaching, with a mini-placement, where you got to be a student teacher for three weeks at an elementary or middle school. I was extremely excited and full of energy heading into this course. It was the only class I was taking that summer semester, and I only worked weekends, so I was fully focussed on it being a success. The course was pass or fail, but had a "highly recommend" category, which gave a grade point average boost when you applied to the Faculty of Education. Being the highly competitive person that I am, I became obsessed with doing everything and more to achieve the "highly recommend". I cruised through the seminars, and was excited for my first day at middle school in a Grade 6 classroom.

Because my main teacher mentor was a vice-principal as well as an English teacher, I split my placement into two classrooms: the English and the science/maths class. My mentor in the science/maths class, and I got along great. However, I did not get along at all well with my English mentor. I made an excellent first impression, but that didn't matter much. On my second day at the school, my English mentor was out of town for a meeting and I was to study under the substitute teacher (sub). When I met the sub, she said, "How would you like to teach the lesson today? The notes are all here."

Now, this was only the second day of what was supposed to be a strictly observational placement, i.e., no teaching. However, I was incredibly eager to teach and hone my skills, and I thought this was a perfect opportunity to build my case for getting the "highly recommend" designation for the course. I agreed to lead the lesson, and it went fantastically well! The kids listened, I asked thought-provoking questions, and I had the substitute teacher in the back of the classroom to give me confidence in classroom management. At the end of the class, the sub said, "Wow, that was great! You're a natural. I'll be sure to leave your mentor a glowing report of what you did today."

I couldn't have been happier. My confidence was buzzing, and when I went back to university that day for a lecture, I bragged to my classmates about how I had just taught a class on my second day. I went on to have a great weekend at work and looked forward to day three of my placement on the Monday.

I walked into the school on my third day with a big grin on my face, greeting my mentor as I walked in. She wiped the smile off of my face pretty quickly. "Where do you get off thinking you can teach my class on your second day of placement?" she curtly asked.

Shocked, I replied, "I don't know – the substitute teacher asked me if I wanted to, and I didn't want to pass on the opportunity."

"Well, I cannot believe you would manipulate a substitute teacher into thinking you were an experienced student teacher! This is an observation-only placement, not a teaching placement!"

"I'm sorry, it won't happen again," I sheepishly replied. Things could only go up from here, I optimistically thought, but I was wrong. She would later tell me that she didn't even want a student teacher, and that she had just failed her last student because they couldn't handle the pressure. My mentor said the previous student had tried too much to be like her and couldn't do it well enough, so they were failed. Also, she said that she didn't care much for my university's education programme, believing the placements happened too early so the students were inexperienced coming into the classroom. I knew she was referring to me. She said she much preferred the way the university she went to ran their programme. After all these comments, I should have requested a transfer, but I was determined to turn things round and get the recommendation.

When I got my first evaluation, it was not good. I got a lot of three out of fives, and even a few two out of fives. In the comments, my mentor had written, "Jason needs to tone down his enthusiasm." This angered me, as I thought I was doing well and that we had buried the substitute teacher day behind us.

Part of the placement involved visiting other classrooms, and my favourite class to visit was a Grade 7 social studies class. The teacher was awesome, and ran a much different classroom than my mentor. When I visited the social studies class on the day I got my evaluation, the teacher asked me what was wrong. I told him about my mark and the comments, and he pulled me aside and said, "Jason, that is complete bullshit. You need enthusiasm as a teacher if you want to truly connect and have fun with kids. Don't let this bring you down." I didn't know at the time, but this uplifting conversation would eventually get me in a lot of trouble later.

I was determined to work on the criticism I had been given. I focussed on my classroom management skills, observed my mentor, took detailed notes and toned down my enthusiasm. On my last day, the Grade 6 children had to write their Provincial Achievement Tests (PATs), and I was assigned to be a scribe for two pupils with learning challenges.

The PAT is a timed test, and the two students I was assigned to needed all the time they could get, so it was important that we started promptly. As we walked to our room to do the test, one boy said he had forgotten his calculator, so we had to go back to get it as this was the Math PAT. Already late, we rushed into the room that was supposed to be empty for us, but there was a boy and an educational assistant in the room folding towels. The boy couldn't help being noisy, and my two students, who were already late starting their test, were struggling to focus on the exam. I was getting stressed out, and I asked the educational assistant how much longer they would be. She took offence at this and left the room. Bewildered, I shook it off and went on scribing the exam.

The two students took the entire allotted time to write the exam, but we got all of it finished. We quietly went back to the classroom, where the other students were working silently on an English assignment. My mentor rushed over to me and said she would be right back, but she had a vice-principal matter to attend to. Not feeling overly confident having to monitor the entire class alone, I went to my desk and hoped there would be no funny business. The students began chatting as soon as the teacher left the room, which was understandable as they had just finished writing a boring two-hour maths exam and were now expected to work silently on an English assignment. I tried to quiet them down, to no avail. They began asking me questions. They were asking me how old I was, and I was trying to tell them that it was inappropriate at this time to ask such a thing, but they kept shouting out guesses. Right at that moment, my mentor walked into the rowdy classroom, and she was furious. "I told you to work silently at your desks! Now quiet down!" She rushed me aside and asked, "What the hell is going on? When I left, it was silent, and now they're asking you about your age? Unacceptable." Then she said, "Oh, and here's your final review." Now, I was pretty shaken, having just being yelled at and put down, so I should have put my evaluation away and looked at it at home when I was calmer. But I didn't. I decided to read it and look at the mark. I was extremely disappointed. I thought I had progressed as I had focussed on the feedback from the first evaluation, but my mark was actually worse. I had passed the placement, but I had no four out fives, and now I had an extra two out of five on classroom management.

Fuming, I wanted some answers as to why my mark was so low. So, I asked my mentor, "Why is my mark here in the twos and threes? What wasn't I doing?"

"Well, I'm not going to change your mark now!" she replied.

"I'm not asking you to. I'm asking for more feedback. Like, why do I have a two for classroom management?"

"Well, today is a perfect example of that, is it not!?" I really didn't think this was fair, and we argued about it for a few more minutes in a heated conversation. I left the classroom disgruntled, and headed to the university for the programme's last lecture.

After the lecture, I told my professor what had happened. She told me, "Sometimes you get a teacher that you just don't vibe with. I wouldn't worry about it, Jason. You passed the class and you're ready for your next placement. I'm confident you'll have a better time next go-round." This made me feel better, and I went into the weekend feeling okay about everything. Little did I know, while my professor and I were talking, she had a voicemail on her phone from my mentor — she wanted to change my grade to a fail.

The next day I went to the gym, and while I was there, I got a phone call from my professor, who asked me to meet her at her office in an hour.

I was extremely nervous. *What could this be about*, I thought? When I arrived, my professor said she had been pleading my case all morning.

"What case?" I asked. She said that my mentor wanted to fail me, which would result in me not being able to take the course again or get into the Faculty of Education. I was shaking, and asked her why my mentor was doing this. My professor said I had broken the code of conduct I had signed at the start of the semester. Confused, I asked her what she was talking about. She cited section 3.4 of the code of conduct: "… student must not challenge a teacher's assessment abilities." I was distraught, and said I didn't do this at all — I was merely asking for additional feedback. She said my mentor took it as a challenge of her assessment ability and wrote me up for it, and also cited that I was rude to an educational assistant — which I thought was absolute garbage. I began to tell my professor that I was not the only person in the school that thought my mentor was wrong about me. I asked if the other teachers I had worked with had any say in my evaluation, and told her how the Grade 7 social studies teacher thought that my enthusiasm was great, and that I shouldn't have been marked poorly because of it. My professor frowned and said, "Unfortunately Jason, I'm going to have to mark that down. You just broke the code of conduct in front of me." Bewildered, I asked her to explain. She cited section 5.4 of the code of conduct: "… student teacher will not discuss other teachers with other staff unless said teacher is present."

I was beginning to get very emotional at this point, and my professor tried to calm me down. She said that she had been fighting for me with the administration all morning to get a "pass not recommend", which meant I had passed the class but would have to retake the course if I wanted to get into the Faculty of Education. I was in disbelief. All semester I had been fighting for the high recommendation, and now I wasn't going to get any recommendation. I told my professor that maybe I wasn't cut out for teaching. I pointed out of her office window to the business building and said, "Maybe I'd be better suited over there." She said I would do great in sales and business, but that I shouldn't necessarily give up on becoming a teacher just yet. She reassured me that in a year I would be more mature and more ready to retake the course. I was still quite disgruntled; I left her office thanking her for fighting for me, but I was crushed inside. I decided a few weeks later that I was going to give business studies a try and changed my major from English to general business, but still combined with the education degree, even though I wasn't so sure about becoming a teacher anymore.

As mad as I was about the whole situation, I am grateful today for the adversity, as it made me grow and change as a person. I was determined to shrug it off and begin the fall with a new attitude, ready for a new set of five classes. I spent the rest of that summer working, but was to find challenges there as well.

4

NEW MAN

While I was enjoying my time at the sports bar, I was starting to have arguments with some co-workers. James was working with the bar now, and I followed him and mirrored everything he did. Some of the other bartenders didn't care for the way James split up tips, however. The traditional way is to split it equally at the end of every night. James' method was to split it up three times through the night, every time someone's shift was over. This way of splitting up tips was advantageous to both him and me because we were regularly the closers and customers regularly tipped more at the end of the night. Management didn't intervene at all, so it went on like this for months.

One shift in the summer, James was not working, but I was closing. My co-worker, who was pregnant at the time, told me at the beginning of the shift that we were going to split tips the original way, not the James way, that night. I got in an argument with her about it. During the middle of the shift, she accused me of pocketing tips (not putting them in the community jar); our manager came over and sent me home for the night. I was furious, because I felt I hadn't done anything wrong. I was, however, in the wrong for getting in an argument with a pregnant senior co-worker, which I now realize.

Our general manager Marty had a chat with me the next day. Marty said my co-workers didn't trust me anymore, and me working there would result in a hostile environment. He said I could work at the company's sister country bar. I took the alternative role, but began looking for a new job immediately, as the country bar was in a bad location and not doing well. I had a trip to Arizona coming up and, before I left town, I applied for a porter position at a place called Duncan's Pub. I thought I was more than qualified for the position, but I saw it as an opportunity to one day become a bartender at the best bar in town.

The Organization

My trip to Arizona had a long backstory. It was a follow-up trip to my trip to Ecuador in 2015, which in itself was a follow-up from when I went to an all-day leadership seminar in high school with my teacher Kevin. Someone had decided at the last minute not to attend the seminar, and Kevin chose me as the replacement because I had donated 52 cans of food for a school food drive.

Why I participated in the food drive is a story in itself. When I sustained a concussion in hockey in 2014, I was left not being able to do very much – watching TV hurt, exercising hurt and even reading hurt. But listening to things was okay. I was bored of listening to music, so I put on a Tony Robbins audiotape I hadn't heard before; it was about the sixth human need of contribution. Robbins tells a story from when he had absolutely nothing. He was broke, out of shape and down to his last $10 bill. He went for a walk on the beach and came across an all-you-can-eat buffet dinner and decided to spend his last dollar on a meal. When he went inside, he noticed a small boy having dinner with his mother. The boy was so polite and courteous to his mother, pulling her chair out for her, etc., that Tony decided to tell the boy how nice he was. He said, "It's so nice of you to take your young lady on a date like this!"

"I'm not on a date. This is my mother. She's buying," he replied.

"No, I think, being the gentleman you are, you'll be paying." And Tony slapped his $10 bill on the table.

The boy said, "I can't take this, sir."

To which Tony replied, "Yes you can, it's a gift," and Tony then walked out the door.

Tony said he never felt more fulfilled in his life. Seeing the smile on that boy's face erased all the hunger and pain he was feeling. He said, "When you give when you have nothing left to give, that's when you're rich." He then went to his apartment, and a cheque for $3,000 was waiting for him from a friend who had borrowed money from him years ago, but Tony had never expected him to pay it back. This money was all Tony needed to get back on his feet; he is now a multi-million-dollar philanthropist and a world-renowned life coach.

At the end of the tape, Robbins implored listeners to set aside an amount of your income that you can gift, no matter what. Whether it's 5, 10 or 15 per cent, the key is to make it automatic. This is called your "Contribution Fund", and it is there so you always have money on hand to give.

I was immediately inspired, so in my concussed state, I rounded up every dollar I had and counted them. I had $520 in total, and had decided that 10% was my number. So, at 7pm on a Sunday night in October, I asked my mom if she would take me to the grocery store so I could buy some cans for the school food drive. She refused because it was too late in the evening, so I walked to the grocery store and bought 52 cans of food.

The annual leadership seminar is for kids that are working towards a goal for either their community or for something international. Motivational speakers talk, performers entertain, and other guests share their story on what it means to be a global citizen. Kids from kindergarten to Grade 12 attend this jam-packed event. At the event there was a draw for teachers, with the grand prize being an all-expenses-paid service and educational trip for a teacher and three students to Ecuador. Kevin put his name in the draw and, out of the thousands of teachers that put their name in the draw, he was called. I was ecstatic for him. Nobody, in my opinion, deserved it more than him. On the bus ride home, I told him that he shouldn't worry about considering me for the trip, as many other students deserved the opportunity. He said he was going to run an application process to decide who would go.

I was always shy about trying new things, and I wasn't much of an outdoors person. I hated getting dirty, and despised bugs. For these reasons, and because I didn't think I deserved to go, I decided not to apply for the Ecuador trip. But my favourite teacher Greg pulled me aside one day after class and convinced me to apply. He said, "You'll never regret travelling. Even if it's a bad experience, you always grow and learn from it. You should really consider applying to Kevin's trip." It was the last day to apply, so I hurried to finish my application. As I was writing it, I got a message from Kevin that said, "Are you sure you're not interested in Ecuador? I need to know asap, because if you don't want the spot, I'll give it to someone else." I was thrilled to be someone he had in mind, and told him he'd have my application on his desk in the morning.

The trip to Ecuador was fantastic. We worked on a water project, and dug a channel and laid pipe for a water duct. I made a lot of friends, and learned so much about being a global citizen and how to be a good leader. The trip facilitators were really impressed with me on the trip, and when it was over the organization offered me a spot on an invite-only follow-up trip in Arizona that focussed on facilitation techniques. Only two groups of 25 people get invited each year, and out of hundreds of kids.

In Arizona, I made a lot of friends who I still connect with today. We learned so much there —over the 12 days, I filled an entire notebook. I was full of energy, but I focussed on channelling that energy internally; I did not want to come across too intense as I had a few months previously at my Education 1000 placement. I wanted to soak everything in and not get into trouble, like I had at the placement and at work. I looked at the trip as a fresh start.

We learned a lot about social justice and about being a global citizen. I found the programming incredibly useful as a potential future teacher. The facilitators also really liked my leadership and listening skills, which I worked on all week. When I got home, I got a phone call from the organization about *another* trip. This one was on international leadership training, and would involve building a school. They said I was the number one candidate out of all the participants on the Arizona trip; it was another invite-only project, where only a few dozen people get the opportunity to go. This one was to Tanzania, Africa. I was thrilled for the opportunity, so I said yes. It was a $5,000 trip, but I had all year to fundraise for it.

I had also just heard back from Duncan's Pub – I had rocked the interview and was given the job. With a new, well-paid position, I was determined to raise the $5,000 all by myself. That September, I had new classes, a new job and a unique opportunity to further my experience of the world. I was reeling with excitement – on top of the world, again – going into that fall semester.

5

WORLD CRASHING

I absolutely loved my job at Duncan's Pub. It was the most professional job I had ever had, and I really liked the staff. It was basically a nightclub on the weekends, and women came out in droves. I picked up a lot of numbers, but I was so busy I never got to follow up because I had to work every weekend. The shifts were long, too. I would start at 7pm and not get off most nights until after 4am. I was making over $200 a night in tips. It was insane to be making that much money, but the hours were insane too. I'd work one five-hour shift on a Wednesday morning, to take in the shipments of liquor, and then two nine-hour shifts on the weekend. So, I was working over 20 hours a week and taking five classes.

I didn't know it at the time, but this was called the hypomanic stage of my bipolar I disorder diagnosis. Everyone around me thought I just had high energy and was super-productive, because I was getting good grades and doing an excellent job at work. Little did I, or anyone else for that matter, know that I was headed down a dark path, which would take a year to recover from.

I thought my job was going well. After New Year's Eve, I worked at the company staff party as the lead porter. At 19, this was a great responsibility, but my boss thought I was killing it on the job. The shift was a mammoth 12 hours, starting at 5pm and ending at 5am. For some reason, the bartenders didn't get paid wage because they were "volunteers", but my boss paid the support staff (me) over $100. This really upset my co-workers, and they seemed to blame me for it, which was completely unfair. However, I did make almost double what they did that night – I walked out with just over $500 in tips because I was tipped out from three different sections of the bar instead of one. I thought I had earned it, but my co-workers were jealous and began to hate me after that shift.

About a week later, my boss pulled me aside and introduced me to our CEO, who was in town. My boss told him how proud he was of me and what a good job I was doing. My boss also casually mentioned that I was going to begin training as one of the youngest bartenders in the company's history. I was thrilled, and couldn't wait to get my training underway. It was a breeze because I remembered all the tricks of the trade James had taught me at the sports bar. As such, I was very cocky. My confidence was at a level ten, and as soon as I started bartending, I acted like a king – and my co-workers hated it. They hated that I had been promoted so fast – they didn't care that I had previous experience – and they despised that I was in the same position as them, taking their shift hours and their tip money.

My co-workers were also furious when they learned I had booked my birthday off, despite it falling on a busy Friday night. They didn't care that I had booked it off three months in advance; they were annoyed because my replacement wasn't as good at the job. I could tell something was up, because my assistant manager was rude to me as I was celebrating with my friends at the bar. My co-workers were also pretty curt with me. I left to go to another bar because they were bumming me out. I shrugged it off as nothing, and figured it would be water under the bridge the next day at work. I was very wrong.

The next day, I arrived at work about a half-hour early to get a bite to eat before my shift. My friend, who was the other porter, was there early too. He sat beside me and said, "Hey Jason, I need to tell you something. Last night, the bartenders really laid into you, saying a bunch of awful stuff in the post-shift meeting to management."

"What were they saying?" I replied.

"They were saying how you're all big-headed now that you've got bartending shifts. They also said some stuff about you wanting to cheat customers or something. Just thought you'd want to know." I thanked him; I had an idea about who led the charge on this slandering. There was one bartender who was a real phoney – he acted as though he liked me but had talked behind my back before. I was determined to confront him that night. I walked past him on my way to the employee area, and he gave me a big smile and said hello. I curtly said hello back, thinking I would lay into him later – but I never got the chance.

When I was walking away from the staff area to start my shift, the general manager and assistant manager blocked me and said, "Jason we need to talk." They fired me on the spot. They said, "Jason, you will not be working tonight, nor will you be working with Duncan's Pub ever again. There has been a breach of trust between you and the bartending staff, and we are going to have to let you go." Bewildered, I asked them to explain what I had specifically done. They said I had been talking about cheating customers. I told them that this couldn't have been further from the truth, but they said they had to trust their senior staff, and the senior staff wanted me gone. But they did say they'd pay for the meal I had just had, which was *oh so kind of them*. I stormed out of the building, and haven't set foot in it since.

I was quite distraught at this moment, so I called up my good friend Dylan and asked if I could come over. At his place, I explained what had happened and smoked a lot of weed with him. He couldn't believe it either, but it didn't matter. The real problem was that I was only about halfway towards saving towards my trip for Africa, and I now had no job. I began working on my résumé the next day, and started applying to jobs that week.

Right around this time, I had started engaging in some risky behaviour, specifically around drugs. I had started smoking marijuana regularly that September, but I was also researching other drugs such as psychedelics. I had found "evidence" that they had the power to awaken a person spiritually and that they could change your life. Of course, I found all this evidence on biased, non-science-based websites, but I nonetheless decided to give magic mushrooms a try. With four other friends, we embarked on our "spiritual journey" together. It was a journey all right, but in hindsight, it was really just a glimpse into what mania would be. I was so high that, at one point, I felt like

I was being sucked into another dimension while Pearl Jam's "Save You" was playing on the TV. Luckily, this heightened state only lasted a night, but reflecting on what I wrote in my phone that night and how I behaved, it was a glimpse into what my summer would be at the height of my mania.

Before I became full-on manic, I continued with my hypomanic super-energy. I quickly bounced back from my Duncan's Pub situation and found *two* new jobs.

6

NEW BEGINNINGS

The week after I got fired from Duncan's Pub, I walked into the bar on the university campus, The Jungle, with my résumé and basically got hired on the spot. I was thrilled, but I knew the money wouldn't nearly be as good as it had been at Duncan's Pub, so I set out to find a second job with my aunt at a catering company. With these two jobs, I was able to fundraise for Africa and have some fun on the side, such as going to see Mumford & Sons and U2.

I was not miserable in my new jobs, by any means; I was, however, frustrated at The Jungle, because I wanted it to be like Duncan's Pub. I was bartending now, but the systems they had in place and the way they did business wasn't even close to the professional environment I was used to. I became obsessed with making The Jungle the best bar in town, and this obsession would eventually get on the nerves of management, as I thought I knew everything. At the catering company, things were great. I loved my fellow staff, and the food we got every shift was phenomenal, and it was a nice break from the spotlight of bartending.

I was still taking five classes and working over 20 hours between the two jobs, but I was happy. I felt very productive, and I was doing well in my business classes. I finished the spring semester strongly, and I was determined to get a pass recommend in my second stint of Education 1000 in the summer semester. I still had to work in the summer so I'd have the money to make my final payment on my Africa trip, but I had found a "balance" between work and school that I thought was good.

This time, Education 1000 went without a hitch. I was paired with a fantastic Grade 3 teacher mentor. Also, I had a new professor who was in his final year of teaching and knew a lot about the field of education. I learned so much from these two. I channelled my energy better this time round, and acted as professionally as possible. Something that helped slow me down, however, was sustaining another concussion after falling off of a mountain.

My friends and I had decided to hike Turtle Mountain. It was an eight-hour total hike, and I wasn't much of an experienced hiker, and I compounded this with the bad choice of smoking weed on the ascent. While the weed "heightened my senses", it nonetheless made me slower and more careless. After peaking the mountain, my friend Ross thought it would be a good idea to go off the path and "scramble" back down; I boldly agreed to follow. It didn't take me long to find a slippery area, and I went tumbling head over heels three times before coming to a halt. I was pretty banged up, and my head really hurt. It was a struggle to hike another four hours to the bottom of the mountain, but, with the help of my friends, I made it. I instantly smoked more pot once we got to the car, which probably wasn't the best idea, given that I had sustained a head injury. I went to the emergency room the next day and was diagnosed with a concussion.

My professor and my mentor were very accommodating, but I do think having concussion helped me pass my placement because it slowed me down. I got my pass recommend, allowing me to apply to the Faculty of Education in the future.

Right around the end of the placement, I made my last payment for the trip to Africa. I was very proud that I had raised the $5,000 all on my own. Also, I had my energy back, and channelled it into work at my two jobs to raise some extra money for the trip.

A few weeks after the placement, on Canada Day, I made a decision that may have changed my life forever.

PART II

MANIA

7

THE BEGINNING OF THE END

To celebrate Canada's 150th birthday on 1 July 2017, a couple of friends and I decided to expand our drug experiences and try LSD. It was one of the dumbest, most irresponsible things I have ever done in my life, and I believe it was one of the primary factors in my admission to hospital just two months later. We took the LSD at my one friend's house at 4pm. His parents were out of town, but his younger brother, who was in Grade 11, was home to "chaperone" us, so we were at least in a safe environment.

When I took the drug, initially nothing happened. LSD is a psychedelic drug that can take a little while to kick in. We had set the house up to facilitate a great time: we had snacks, concerts to watch, a stereo, and it was a beautiful sunny day. I was sitting outside, staring at the sky, when the drug started to kick in. I was watching clouds form while listening to rock and roll music – it was trippy. After a while, I went into the house to put The Doors concert DVD on. I was absolutely enthralled by the rainbow colours that were reflecting on the blank TV screen from the lamp. I was so set on experiencing the drug, I thought this was the drug playing tricks on me – obviously, it wasn't. While I watched The Doors DVD, I began writing down nonsense about how "this pen is a detachment from my brain", and a whole bunch of gibberish about what I thought was metaphysics. During this experience, I was convinced that "brilliant minds just smartly use psychedelics to reach a higher level of being". I wrote, "We need more spaces in the world to do LSD in."

After journaling non-stop for a few hours, I walked outside to where my friends' brother was and talked with him for a while. My other two friends had left the house to "go exploring". While we were talking – I thought I was being philosophical, but I mostly spoke gibberish – I began hallucinating, and his face began to "melt"; it was as if his face was morphing into something else. It was trippy as hell, and I still have the image in my head to this day.

I finally went home around 2am, after smoking a lot of weed to "calm down" from the LSD. I was still full of energy, so I watched some YouTube videos that were supposed to be trippy while high on LSD in my garage. An hour later, and when I walked out of my garage, I hallucinated again. The street lights looked as if they were cotton balls full of light, like giant spheres of white light. I couldn't believe it was 3am, and I was still feeling the effects of LSD.

I walked into my bedroom to go to bed, but I accidentally saw my reflection in the mirror. The one thing the guy who sold me the LSD said *not* to do was look in a mirror, because your eyes get incredibly dilated when on LSD and it can cause you to freak out. I remember seeing my reflection for just a split second and being terrified. I hated the image of my dilated eyes. Later in my mania, I would be obsessed with my eyes and the dilation of them.

When I had calmed down from seeing my reflection, I journaled for another hour and my writing was all over the place. If anyone else had read it, I think I would have been committed to the hospital sooner. It was evidence of my racing thoughts, grandiose ideas and fast thinking, which are all symptoms of bipolar mania. Finally, at 4am, I hit the pillow and drifted off to sleep. I was working the next day at 2pm, so I slept until about noon. I woke up feeling different, enlightened maybe. In reality, I was stepping into the realms of what is called a manic episode, where one regularly has racing thoughts, rapid speech and a detachment from reality. I thought I felt fine – better than ever, in fact. I remember walking to work and appreciating the nature around me. I was super happy and ready to work. I was also extremely excited about my trip to Africa, which was only a few weeks away. Everything seemed like it was coming together for me and, yet again, I felt like I was on top of the world.

8

ROAD TO AFRICA

Two things I was determined to do after taking LSD was to get a medicinal marijuana card and invest in a marijuana company. I believed in the product, and wanted to get legal, licensed marijuana, so no one could complain about me smoking too much. I went about this by booking an appointment with a "weed doctor". I didn't actually need marijuana for medicinal purposes, so I came up with every ailment that weed could help me with. I told the doctor that I had depression, anxiety, back pain and trouble sleeping. Whether he could tell I was lying or not, it didn't matter. He wrote me a prescription, and I was out the door. I signed up with Aurora Cannabis minutes later on my phone and, within a week, I had my medicinal marijuana card.

I had heard of Aurora from a friend of mine who had a prescription with them. I really liked their packaging, distribution system and product. In my accounting class, we learned how to do a financial analysis of businesses using ratios, equations, etc. I decided I would do the same financial analysis with Aurora. The numbers came out okay, and the stock price was only $2.49 a share as it was only a year old. I was determined to buy shares before I left for Africa, and I actually pressed the "buy" button in the airport, right before we boarded the plane. My obsession with the investment really annoyed my mother, as that and being busy with work meant I still hadn't packed for my trip the day before I was due to leave.

My grandparents came down from up north to wish me well on my trip to Africa, and my grandma helped me pack. Although it was pretty stressful packing for 16 days in one afternoon, I luckily had everything I needed. I had to bartend a wedding the night before I left, and it was a 13-hour shift, so I was absolutely exhausted the next day. My plan was to get dropped off in Calgary the day before my connecting flight to Toronto, so that I could visit my friend Will, who would then drive me to the airport the next morning. My grandparents drove me to Calgary; in hindsight, they should have turned round and taken me home.

On the drive to Calgary, I was definitely showing signs of bipolar mania: rapid speech, racing thoughts and emotional behaviour. I told my grandparents how my dad and I weren't getting along, how I was stressed out at work, and how I was a bit scared to go to Africa. I talked to them about random ideas too – how, one day, I would get a licence to fly a helicopter and maybe own island property in Fiji. I also brought up some touchy subjects about our family and got emotional about them. They dropped me off at Will's place after I had just finished crying, and they both told me they loved me very much. I instantly fell asleep on Will's couch, and woke up rested and less manic. Good thing too, because Will had to go to work for a few hours, leaving me to have dinner with his parents and their friends.

I had a nice dinner and a good chat with Will's family. His mom was the principal at an international school in China, and his stepdad was responsible for recruitment to the school. I treated the dinner like an interview, because, who knows, maybe I would want to teach in China one day. I impressed them so much so that Will's mom said to call her when I graduated. When Will got back, we hung out and played some guitar before I called it a night and went to bed.

I had scheduled in a day in Toronto after my connecting flight so I could catch a Blue Jays game and see the Hockey Hall of Fame. On my way from the Hall of Fame to the ball diamond, I smelled weed and asked the guy it was emanating from if I could have a puff. Flying high, I looked up at the skyscrapers and buildings of Toronto and got ready for the game.

The game was fun, but I was craving more pot after ward. I had a friend I'd met in Arizona who lived in Toronto, so I called him, and we met up after the game. He didn't have any pot though, so I had to take an Uber to an illegal dispensary to get some. We smoked all night with a few other friends, and I told them all about my trip to Africa the next day. One of my friends had some experience of one of the organization's facilitators, and she warned me that she could be challenging to be around and that I should be careful. Being stoned, I didn't pay too much attention to what she way saying. We had a fun night before I took an Uber back to my hotel. I was high as a kite and ready to embark on my journey to Africa the next day.

9

AFRICA

I had a lot of ambitious goals for this trip, and had listed 24 before we even landed and came up with a further 14 by the second day. I had done some research before the trip on speed reading and other accelerated learning techniques by peak performance expert and author, Tim Ferriss. A lot of my goals had to do with my "performance" on the trip. I was convinced that I was walking into an internship-like situation, when I really wasn't. I was called a Leader International, and was the oldest participant on the trip. I was to focus on learning facilitation techniques by shadowing the facilitators.

I was doomed to repeat the same behaviour I exhibited when I took Education 1000 the first time. Then I had been obsessed with getting a "high recommendation"; this time I was obsessed with getting a job with the organization that was running the trip. I wanted to be the youngest part-time facilitator they had ever had. My goal was to be working for them next summer at age 21. This was an unrealistic goal as this organization has incredibly high standards when it comes to who runs and facilitates their trips. Usually, the candidate already has some management or leadership training and a university degree in their back pocket. I was still three years away from graduating, and did not stand a chance of getting a position. But that didn't stop me from being obsessed with the idea.

My time in Africa is well documented, as I ferociously journaled nearly every second of the trip. Over the 16-day experience, I filled a back-to-back 250-page coil notebook, 51 pages in a medium-sized journal and two and a half pocket journals. I also had over two and a half hours of audio journal content, and a few dozen pages of notes written on my phone. I was constantly writing down my thoughts, feelings and ambitions. They can basically be summed up in one word: grandiose. Grandiosity is usually a symptom of the bipolar manic phase, as a person in that state is so elevated they feel anything is possible. And I most definitely did; for example, in one of my journals, I wrote, "YOU WILL ACCOMPLISH ALL YOU WANT IN LIFE BECAUSE YOU ARE SUPERHUMAN." I wrote in the second person a lot – it was like an ongoing conversation with myself that never stopped. I was very excited all the time – in one entry, I describe myself as "literally bouncing with energy and passion". Rambling was very common, and the use of capital letters was everywhere. It was also pretty messy writing at times, as if I couldn't write fast enough.

Insomnia – another symptom of the manic state – was starting to show early on in the trip too. I had so much energy, I frequently went to bed late and woke up early. Most nights I fell asleep between midnight and 3am, and woke between 6am and 8am. The group was set up in tents, and I shared with three other guys. One night, early on in the trip, I couldn't get to sleep at the scheduled 10pm curfew, so I snuck out of my tent with my sleeping bag, pillow and headphones, set up a three-chair bed under the Tanzanian night sky, and stargazed while listening to Roger Waters' *In the Flesh* concert on my phone. We weren't allowed to leave our tents at night for safety reasons, but this act of defiance was the start of a long stretch of rule-breaking by me on the trip. I fell asleep outside; the cold woke me up around 4am and I returned to my tent. It was one of my favourite moments of the trip, and I will never forget the way the night sky and stars looked that peaceful night.

Breaking Rules

I remember the trip fondly, but I also remember being rebellious. Because the group of participants ages ranged from 14 to 20, there had to be a lot of safety precautions and rules. These included:

no leaving the tent at night, which I broke almost immediately; no drinking or smoking, because most of the participants were under age. I broke the no smoking and no drinking rule when we stopped for gas one day about a week into the trip – I purchased a mickey of vodka and paid one of the drivers to buy me a pack of cigarettes. It was the longest stretch of being sober for me since I started drinking and smoking pot a year earlier – and I couldn't handle it anymore.

Imagine your worst hangover and multiply it by ten and you'll have an idea of how I was feeling the day after I drank the vodka. I drank the entire mickey in one night after sneaking out of my tent. I masked the hangover with the excuse of dehydration, and was able to get out of most of the planned activities. There was no way I was going to move bricks for the school we were building in that condition.

I started smoking cigarettes because I was missing marijuana a lot. I even flirted with the idea of getting one of the drivers to score me some local pot, but my friend (and Masai warrior), Lebohaiti, strongly urged against it because he said it was known for making his people crazy. I figured the quality wouldn't be as good as the medicinal grade stuff I was getting at home, so I opted for cigarettes instead. I was never a smoker, so I only needed about half a cigarette to feel a good buzz, but the night I drank all the vodka I also had four cigarettes, which just added to my misery the next morning.

I could have been sent home from the trip for these offences, but I didn't care as I couldn't take the abstinence from drugs and alcohol any longer. After the hangover passed, I was soon back to my rapid thinking and grandiose goal setting – I was incredibly inspired by the activities of the trip, and was determined that I would change the world.

Changing the World

The organization I was travelling with prides itself on providing meaningful trips for youth. The goal is to have participants coming home feeling confident they can make a positive change in their community and in the world. The facilitators regularly mentioned how we could "change the world," – of course, they meant in small ways and not literally changing the world. In my manic state, I took this message literally, and became seriously obsessed with the idea of changing the world.

I was going to change Africa, North America and the whole world by the time I was 30. I would do this in a multitude of ways. For example, I was going to start the Wegner Ways Corporation, have a #1 ranked podcast, write a dystopian novel, run two charities, get two PhDs, become a teacher, play concerts in a Pink Floyd cover band in Africa for free, and become a world-class musician. All of this would be done within the decade, as I was obsessed with the idea planted in my head by Tony Robbins that "most people underestimate what they can do in a decade", and by my old coach Trevor Hardy's quote, "Success is time used effectively." I wrote in my journal early in the trip, "My success is quantified by the amount of lives I improve", and I was determined to accomplish these massive goals so I could change the world for the better.

These ideas really became prevalent and more common in my journals after the day we went without food. One of the modules on the trip was to experience the same hunger as those in developing nations, so we fasted for an entire day. They fed us mush for breakfast, which I had half a bowl of, and then some lentils and beans for lunch, which I barely picked at because I didn't like it. By 11am, I was already stewing with anger and passion, coming up with ideas to change the world and end world hunger. I knew that the day would be a mental and physical battle, and while my energy was pretty low, my mind was racing.

Thinking about my job with the catering company, I got incredibly angry at the industry as a whole for all the food wasted, and was determined to make a change when I got home. I planned to make my aunt's business a "no-waste catering business", and get the company to allow staff to take more food home. My ideas were flowing, and I continued my quest for solving world hunger with my next idea: getting grocery stores to lower food waste. I believed that if I could get my local grocery store to adopt a no-waste policy, many others would follow.

I also came up with the idea for a corporation called Wegner Ways, which would spread ideas others could action and thereby "change the world". But I wasn't done yet – I also came up with the idea for a charity called "People Feeding People", which would bypass the red tape of giving away leftover food from events and the expired-but-still-edible food from grocery stores. These ideas were mostly expressed in capital letters in my journal, and I figured that I had to accomplish all of these goals to change the world. Failure to achieve these goals was not an option.

By about midday, I was starting to fall deeper into my thoughts. It was a very humbling experience, because I felt like my pain was not even close to what real people in poverty face every day. I wrote in capital letters in my journal, "I DO NOT HAVE ANY PROBLEMS IN MY LIFE", and that this day would be a reference point for my future. I felt like I was very close to breaking.

My hunger and mania was also making me easily annoyed by some of the participants. We were between activities, and I was sitting in the common area journaling when I saw two participants eating a granola bar. Eating was against the rules of the day, and they were bragging about it. They were two of the American participants, and I called them out. I called them "selfish, American pigs", and said, "This is why people around the world hate Americans." This comment was pretty harsh, but I was in a state of complete lack of control. Another American participant told one of the facilitators about my comment and, rightfully so, I got in trouble.

At the time, I was convinced of a quote I had read before the trip by author and inspirational speaker Simon Sinek: "Leaders eat last", so I regularly went in line after everyone else had been served. Many of the people on the trip took more than they ought, so I was left with the scraps. I felt like I had the biggest appetite of the group, so I was steaming mad. On top of all of this, it was my turn to help with the dishes, and I hate doing dishes. The day just kept on getting worse, and I was getting more and more agitated. Even the flies were causing me distress. It seemed like everyone's energy was good but mine, and, as I wrote in my journal, I was "in a full state of agitation".

I was so hungry that all I could do was think, and my brain was on overdrive, continually spiralling into all of these ideas. I really believe this was the tipping point in my mania. As my journaling increased, so did the size of my ideas. I was very agitated and angry, but also inspired. I wrote down that I wanted to "be the next Tony Robbins, Tim Ferris, Trevor Hardy, that changed the world." I wrote, "I have 80 years to change the world", which I found very encouraging at the time. I was beyond certain that all of these plans would work out and happen. I was convinced, ironically, that I could do everything with "holistic pragmatism", i.e., think of all the factors involved and then take pragmatic, realistic steps towards achieving them. My main answer to every doubt any of these grandiose goals triggered was the simple yet powerful question, "Why Not?" Asking "Why Not?" was my excuse for every behaviour and idea I had during my manic episode. It made me think that anything was possible. My anger and passion flowed throughout the day, and my facilitators told me to "take it easy with the rambling".

For one activity, the facilitators made a rule where I couldn't talk and had to communicate with my team non-verbally. This rule was nearly impossible and incredibly frustrating. Trying to get a manic person to stop talking is like trying to get a dog to stop barking. I cheated multiple times, and pushed my team further back in the activity. Tempers flared, and it was quite unpleasant for everyone. However, once we finally broke the fast with a real meal, I started to settle down, and everyone was happy again. The day had been incredibly challenging.

I became obsessed to a fault with some of my new ideas, especially the idea of writing a dystopian novel called *2084*, which (of course) I believed would change the world.

The Novel

The main premise for my novel was that it would be set in a future where the extreme left had finally taken political control after years of the extreme right being been in power. The leader in America was a character named Madame President, a transgender, power-hungry monster who will do anything to get her way. She implements a mandatory, politically correct society that is enforced by the Vocabulary Police. The Vocabulary Police wear dark, rainbow-coloured uniforms, and if someone in society speaks in a politically incorrect manner, they administer mind-controlling drugs to reset their brain to a docile, obedient, non-offensive one.

The other main idea was that everything is controlled by "Society", and Society keeps everyone in line. I had scribbled in my journals things like "SOCIETY MUST ALWAYS KNOW WHERE YOU ARE" and "SOCIETY IS IN CONTROL". Madame President makes marijuana legal across America, but alters the marijuana plants to control everyone's mind so that Society is under her control.

The protagonist was based on me, and he one day offends someone by speaking his mind and gets taken away by the Vocabulary Police and drugged by them. The main character would have a similar backstory to my own, mainly being that he had travelled to Africa in his 20s and learned the Masai warrior way. The main action in the novel would be the main character somehow breaking the spell Madame President had over him and finding his way back to Africa, where he conspires with the African people to fledge a full war on America and overthrow the tyrannical government.

I was convinced that this novel would be a bestseller and that people would absolutely want to read about the "dangers of a politically correct society"; I thought it would be my generation's *1984*. I wrote down that I would have it published within the next ten years and that it would be a masterpiece.

When I started writing *this* book, I realized that it was my frustrations on the trip that had fuelled my ideas for the novel. Basically, everything in the novel was connected to the trip. Everything that was upsetting me on the trip, I magnified into the story. I was trying to write the opposite of my idea of utopia into a novel. For example, my idea for the Vocabulary Police stemmed from people constantly telling me to "watch my words", because they were borderline offensive. And the

Madame President character was a caricature of one of the facilitators on the trip who I was repeatedly clashing with. I was also starting to become paranoid about the government at this time, which is why I was scared of some official forcing mind-controlling drugs on me. I didn't want to conform, I wanted to be rebellious – hence the main character's modus operandi of government overthrow and war.

It was really all quite silly in hindsight, but my notes provide an eye-opening look into how my thoughts were being formed and what was shaping them.

The Band

In addition to the novel, I was going to write a concept album that would have similar themes to the novel. Basically, I wanted to be the next Pink Floyd and write my own *The Wall* masterpiece, as I was obsessed with that album. The idea of a Pink Floyd cover band had probably been in my head since seeing one a few months earlier. My plan was that, as the popularity of my cover band grew, I would seed in original tunes that sounded like Pink Floyd, which would get the band public exposure. I was so optimistic about this band that I was certain that, by age 30, I would have launched a tour and sell out stadiums globally, starting in Tanzania.

All these ideas meet the definition of grandiose. To start with, I am really not a very good singer or guitar player, and I hardly knew any other young musicians who would want to follow my crazy vision. The odds of me ever becoming a world-class musician on top of all my other big plans was simply ridiculous. I also wanted to play Pink Floyd's *The Wall* in Tanzania for free, which is also absurd as it's one of the most expensive shows ever to be put on by a band, and I don't think Pink Floyd's popularity is exactly huge at this time in Africa. My main objective was to get on Roger Waters' radar, because I thought I was the chosen one to continue his legacy of the remarkable political music he is known for. Plus, I wanted to interview Waters for my other crazy idea of running and hosting a number-one ranked podcast called "Wegner Ways".

The Podcast

The podcast idea was basically a rip-off of "The Tim Ferriss Show", which has record-breaking numbers of downloads. I wanted to take Ferriss's concept of interviewing top performers about their specific daily routines, strategies and life advice and make it my show. I listed in my journal over 50 people I wanted to interview, such as Prime Minister Justin Trudeau. As I have a friend who was then working for Trudeau, I thought it would be "easy" to interview him and get my podcast on the map. As much as I thought I had everything planned out to a tee, most of the people on my list are ludicrous. For example, I planned to get Leonardo DiCaprio on the show and have him meet one of my friends from the trip, because he's our favourite actor. I thought this was possible because, as I constantly repeated to myself, "Why not?"

Education

One of the main focusses of my goals was education. I wanted to get PhDs in both English and Education, and I wanted to change the school curriculum in both North America and in Africa. I wrote that I wanted to get a PhD so I could "say whatever the hell I wanted", as that's what I thought the main perk of having a PhD was. I felt that I could one day change the curriculum in both places to have a better, more "pragmatic" approach. I realize, in hindsight, that I just wanted to create a curriculum that would result in more people like me.

I was determined that I would come back and teach in Tanzania. I even priced it out, figuring that I would basically break even as a teacher in Tanzania but could make money through investments. It was an idea that many shot down, so I kept it to myself for most of the trip, secretly dreaming of having my own classroom in the school we were building.

The Charity

In addition to my education goals, I wanted to create a charity called Homo Sapiens First, which would basically be like George Costanza's "Human Fund" from the 1990s TV show *Seinfeld*. I figured I could create a charity that would help people and people only. It was a *very* vague goal, but I was on a roll with making goals, so that didn't concern me.

The Corporation

I figured I had struck gold with my ultimate goal of a corporation, which – of course – I thought would change the world – a perfect example of my grandiosity. I planned to create a corporation that would be all about outsourcing, but treating people well at the same time – for example, minimum-wage factories, but with excellent benefits. It would be called something like "People First", and the whole idea would be about treating employees like gold. The corporation would build business models that made sense, and put the employees before the business. I ranted about this idea for over 30 minutes one morning in an audio journal, and was crying to myself, "I have limited time. I can't do all of this, but this may be my greatest gift to the world." I was certain the "invisible plan" was there, and I just had to write it down. I repeated, "My success is not determined by any monetary amount. It's determined by how many lives I change." I was beyond certain that building business models that put employees first would change the world. I was really emotional about this because I thought it would help children.

The children we met on the trip made me think a lot about how different the lives of kids in Tanzania are from the lives of those in Canada. I wanted Tanzanians to have the same opportunities that Canadian kids had, i.e., access to clean water, schools to attend and nutritious food to eat. I said in that same audio journal entry, "There shouldn't be a Third World and a First World – it should be One World! We're homo sapiens first, not black or white or any other race."

Changing the world became my main objective, and I was determined to do it in a decade. I calculated – to the hour – how much time I had until I turned 30 to accomplish my big five goals of writing a dystopian novel, becoming a world-class musician, having a number one-ranked podcast, finishing my Education degree, and building and running a corporation. Factoring in time spent eating and sleeping, I had 57,675 hours of productivity to accomplish all my goals. This number seemed so big, my plans seemed achievable to me. Tony Robbins' saying of "Most people underestimate what they can do in a decade" rang through my head daily. I did have some fear I wouldn't accomplish my goals, but I convinced myself that these were "false fears" and that, because I was on the path to becoming "superhuman", my goals would all fall into place eventually.

The 10 per cent

My ambitious thinking was not well received by some people on the trip, including the facilitators. Nobody was trying to put me down, but they were trying to keep me grounded. I recorded one of my conversations with a facilitator, where I explained the corporation idea. I rambled on for about ten minutes, not letting him barely get a word in, and he basically just humoured me, but others didn't. I had learned about the Pareto principle through a Tim Ferriss podcast, which basically states that 80 per cent of consequences (which I translated as my problems) come from 20 per cent of causes (which I translated as the people around me). I began to identify that about 10 per cent of the people on the trip were causing 90 per cent of my stress by shooting down my ideas, challenging me and pissing me off. I became obsessed with this 10 per cent, and developed what I called the "invisibility shield", where I basically imagined that this 10 per cent had the plague and were to be avoided at all costs.

In my journals, I wrote excessively about the 10 per cent, and believed they would be my demise. I continued to repeat to myself that I only had a decade to accomplish my goals, and that I couldn't let anyone or anything stand in my way, as my goals were too important. I must have appeared a lunatic to most of the participants on the trip, with my rambling speeches and outlandish plans, pacing back and forth and recording my audio journals. Most people on the trip had good intentions, and wanted what was best for me, but because I was manic, I was extraordinarily obstinate and narrow-minded. I had a lot of plans for when I got back to Canada, and the idea of the 10 per cent enemy would extend to those back home as well.

Need for Freedom

Because I had so many world-changing projects on the go, I knew when I got home from Africa I would need some space to accomplish my goals. I didn't think my parents would support me in all my goals, simply because they hadn't experienced Africa. Having seen the poverty and the willingness of people to improve their lives, I was convinced that the world could change, and that I would be the one to change it. I thought I had specific, actionable goals, but I really didn't – they were bombastic, mega-goals. Nevertheless, I was convinced that I needed a new space back home to do all my work, so I decided I would move out of my parents' place.

I had always lived at home for financial reasons and convenience. I had made up my mind, however, that it was selfish to be a financial burden on my parents any longer, particularly as I was going to become a master in investing. I already had a mutual fund that was performing modestly, and I was confident that my marijuana stock would make me rich. I wrote in one of my journals, "Money is no issue because I am a master investor." Money through investing would fuel all my goals, I said to myself. I was also planning on working three jobs when I got home. When I calculated it was affordable to move out, I got excited. I was excited about the freedom to smoke pot, bring girls over and work on my massive goals. In my phone notes, I have an extremely detailed plan of how I was going to move out, where I would draw the money from and who I would move in with. It was one of the first things I told my parents when I landed home in Canada, which was almost earlier than planned.

Last Strike Behaviour

During one of my regular nightly meetings with the facilitators, I was told to step up my game, to stop leaving my tent after curfew, to stop being late for activities, to stop wearing headphones so much, and to stop talking about alcohol to the other participants. They said this was my last strike, as I had already been warned twice, and I was about to be written up and sent home. I was very frustrated at this because, the way I saw it, I couldn't sleep so early in the night due to insomnia; I was only ever a minute late because I had important journaling to do; I wore headphones all the time so I would keep my mouth shut, because I was "irritating" people; and I had had maybe one conversation about alcohol because I was asked about it, but the facilitators overheard it. In my opinion, the other participants had free rein to say whatever they wanted, but I had to unfairly follow more rules. In hindsight, they had a point – leaving my tent and being late set a bad example; having my headphones on all the time made me appear standoffish; and talking about alcohol to minors was obviously unprofessional, given that I was in a leadership role. But I was manic, so didn't see it that way. I felt like it was another attack on me by the lead facilitator – aka Madame President, the tyrannical monster.

Nonetheless, I was on my best behaviour for the rest of the trip, and managed to made it to the last day.

10

HEADING HOME

I was determined to return to Africa in five years, and I had told my *rafikis* (friends) that I would be back by 2022. Although Africa already felt like a second home, when I was there, I was beyond homesick. I had told my mom to make sure to bring my herbalizer (marijuana device) and medicinal marijuana with her when she picked me up; I could not wait for that moment of ultimate satisfaction after two and a half long weeks of being without marijuana.

On the plane ride home, I started to compose three extremely long emails to the important people in my life who would want to know how my trip had gone. One was to my former teacher mentor from Education 1000, one to my professor from Education 1000, and one to the superintendent of the local school district. In the one to the superintendent, I wrote, "It's pretty hard to steady my mind with all the amazing lessons and reflections from my experience in Tanzania." I bragged about learning how to speed read and talked about being a teacher that develops "super-learners". I ended with, "I know for a fact that I will return to Tanzania and work with the community again."

Surprisingly, she replied to my email; she wrote that it was "… great to hear from you. It certainly sounds like you had a very enlightening and enriching experience. Let me know when you are doing your next practicum [placement] with our district and I'll stop by and touch bases." I was thrilled with this response, and truly felt that my emailing prowess would advance my career.

To travel from Tanzania to my hometown involves nearly 27 hours of air travel and a two-and-a-half-hour drive. In my layover in Toronto,

I seriously contemplated getting an Uber to drive me to a dispensary to buy some marijuana edibles for the plane ride from Toronto to Calgary. Given that I only had a two-hour layover, this idea was absurd. Instead, I stayed at the airport and ate a massive amount of Wendy's hamburgers.

Although I should have been tired from all the air travel, I was quite energetic on my flight from Toronto to Calgary. The couple sitting next to me on the plane started up a conversation with me based on the oversized safari hat I was wearing. They were lucky enough to have me talk their ears off for the three-hour flight from Toronto to Calgary, hearing all about my trip and a lot about my book idea. I had written 46 pages of notes on that day alone. They seemed interested, but I am sure they were just humouring me. I told them I would give them a copy of my novel, so they gave me their email. Hopefully, they're not disappointed reading a copy of this book instead of the masterpiece novel *2084* I pitched them.

When I landed in Calgary, my parents happily greeted me. It was the longest stretch I'd ever been away from them, and I was happy to see them too. I was heartbroken to learn my mom had "forgotten" the herbalizer and medicinal marijuana. "She had one job," I recall

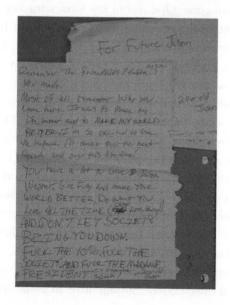

thinking. It didn't feel like a very long drive, however, because I talked the entire two and a half hours. I told them all about the trip, especially about the lead facilitator (Madame President). I remember narrowing in and focussing on my frustrations of the trip more than anything. Thinking back on it, my parents were somewhat concerned but they chalked it up to just being excited about being home and the experiences I had just had. We stopped to pick up pizza before we went home, and it felt like an eternity before we got our food. I was craving marijuana so bad that I got into an argument with my mother about it when my dad exited the car to get the food. I was angry she didn't bring the herbalizer, but she assured me we would be home in ten minutes and that I could smoke up then.

As soon as we got home, I made a beeline for the shed where my pot was stored – I didn't even say hello to my pets. I immediately smoked up, and smoked up a lot. I had my medicinal-grade marijuana, and life was good. Five minutes later, my dad came out and angrily asked me why I couldn't wait until after we had dinner to smoke up. I explained how it had been 16 days of sobriety and that I was merely doing it while he was washing up for dinner. "*Hakuna matata*," I said.

We sat down for dinner, and I was stoned out of my mind. My eyes were bloodshot red, and I was barely formulating sentences as I mowed down greasy pizza. My dad was so disgusted he left the room and ate his dinner downstairs. I don't think I had ever disappointed him so much in my entire life. But I didn't care at that moment. I was actually happier than I'd been in weeks. I had to eat dinner relatively fast because my friend Ross was on his way to pick me up for a softball game. It was the championship final, and I had made it back just in time.

The Championship Game

I was stoned, but had a lot of energy due to the mania, and was ready to play some softball. I was telling my friend Ross all about the trip, and when I arrived to meet the rest of the team, I greeted them in

Swahili and said a few other phrases to them while I told them about my trip.

One of my teammates told me, "Speak fucking English, Jason, you're in Canada." We got into a bit of an argument over that, but I went on talking about my trip to whoever would listen. A few humoured me, but one said, "Listen Jason, no one really cares about your trip, we've got a game to play." I was getting tired, so I shut my mouth finally and got ready for the game. I don't remember much of the game as I continued to smoke weed and have a few drinks. I remember having a "micro-nap" in the bottom of the last inning and being woken up because I was on deck. I did ten push-ups to wake my body up, and was dialled in when I went into the on-deck circle. The game was tied, and there was one out with a runner on third. Either my friend ahead of me would win the game, or it would be up to me. He grounded out to second, and the runner stayed at third. It was up to me to win the game. I wasn't nervous. I had been here before in my minor-league days and, as I was pretty stoned and a little drunk too, my confidence levels were pretty high. I stepped into the batter's box, ready to win the game. First pitch was a ball. The second one, a strike. I was ready to swing on the third pitch, and I drilled the ball past the first baseman and ran to first. The winning run ran home, and we won the game.

It was a surreal feeling – it felt like we had just won the World Series (which was most likely due to the drugs and alcohol). We partied all night at the diamond, and I had a lot of fun. It was the perfect homecoming for me, aside from the fact that I had really upset my dad. Our relationship would continue to be strained over the next few weeks as my condition continued to deteriorate.

I was becoming full-blown manic. After 20 days of full-blown mania, I was finally hospitalized.

11

FULL-BLOWN MANIA

The Handout

As a caveat, I should mention that the organization I travelled with did supply a "Welcome Your World Traveller Home" handout, but I didn't read it. My mom asked me to, but I was swamped when I got home from the trip. In the handout, it said the trip was a "life-changing experience", and that travellers "often return home feeling empowered and ready to take what they've learned and turn it into action." However, it also said that the trip experience could evoke everything from "excitement, all the way to frustration." This described me perfectly – I was experiencing both extremes. I was incredibly excited to change the world, but very frustrated because it seemed like everyone around me was thinking small. The handout also mentions that "feeling emotionally 'displaced' after returning home is commonly referred to as 'reverse culture shock,' and is completely normal." Reverse culture shock didn't seem a strong enough way of describing how I felt on coming home – it was more like a reverse culture earthquake. The handout said that "support is more valuable than ever", but I was only looking for support for my big ideas. Lastly, the handout said, "The real journey starts when the students arrive home," and that could not have been a more accurate statement.

First Days Home

On my second day home, I was still scribbling like a madman in my pocket journals. From that day alone, I have 49 pages of notes. They're all over the place, but I did write, "Culture shock is a thing, readjust well." I tried to readjust by going for a walk with my mom and dog. I wasn't high, but I sure seemed like it. My thoughts were coming at me a mile a minute as I was telling my mom all about how I would change the world. I asked her what she would do if money was no object. She told me how she always wanted to run a greenhouse and teach people how to garden. I vowed I would help with this, and then I told her about all my business plans. I was also frank with her and told her about my LSD experience, which shocked her. She never thought I would touch hard drugs like LSD. I never viewed psychedelics as hard drugs, however – I thought they were a tool that unlocked the brain. In reality, they are a tool that can break the brain.

I journaled that day, while stoned, about how "micro dosing", or taking small amounts of psychedelics, could give my performance at school an edge. I did some (extremely biased) research on micro dosing psychedelics, and it seemed like a great idea. A few other thoughts I noted down included Tony Robbins' phrase, "Don't be a master in minor things." I flipped that quote on its head and wrote, "Be an Expert in ALL THINGS. Be brilliant because WHY NOT." I wrote that I could "be a master in English, psychology and neuroscience." The idea of being an "expert in all things" would be a theme throughout my mania, as I couldn't decide what I wanted to be. I would later say I wanted to have a PhD in Everything. My thoughts were swirling, but I believed that journaling and smoking more pot would help. It did not, and I just continued the descension into more rabbit holes and random thoughts.

Volunteering

Another idea I had when I first got home was to find a place to volunteer. I started brainstorming in an audio journal (I have a lot of these). "Maybe I'll be Tim Ferriss's personal assistant, i.e., shadow my hero. Me and Tim will go to the moon! I don't know, anything can happen!" But, instead of flying to San Francisco to track down the famous writer of the *The 4-Hour Work Week*, I decided to try and find somewhere in town to volunteer.

I found a church thrift store downtown that gave me a form to fill out, and I gave "enthusiastic" answers.

Time Commitment – "Not sure yet, to be honest, I'm trying to find the right organization for me and my passions."

What school or organization do you require volunteer hours for – "Life."

Reasons for volunteering – I put an emphatic check mark next to all the choices.

Interested in doing – I also put an emphatic check mark alongside all these choices too, and wrote, "Everything and anything you need!"

Creativity – "I am a writer."

By the end, the form was covered with long, detailed and scattered answers. However, I never handed in the form – I was just too busy.

In another audio journal, which I recorded while I was under the influence of marijuana, I described myself as "a student of the world", and said, "People need to destigmatize psychedelics." I went on to say "Hi" to my future self, which started a one-way conversation. "How ya doing, future Jason?! Man, things are great. Life is an elephant, and I'm just the rider, riding its highs and lows. What if I changed my career every ten years? Knowledge compounds, so I would be just getting smarter and smarter throughout each decade. You can make a positive change on a massive scale. WWx. Wegner Ways everywhere! Wow, yeah, I'm moving at 100 miles an hour, but my brain thinks at 100 miles an hour. My gosh, it's nice having a brain that I understand how it works!"

The mind working at 100 miles per hour is a good representation of what my mania was like. I was in my parents' place when I made this particular recording, and I was becoming paranoid, most likely due to the "medicine". I explained in it how I was afraid that my parents would walk in on me making a voice recording or talking to myself, and think I was crazy. But I felt like I was note-taking too much in journals, so I thought that audio journaling was the better route for recording my brilliant thoughts.

Moving Out

My main priority when I got home from Tanzania was to move out of my parents' place. I was looking at two possible places: one to share with my friend Jurgy, his girlfriend and two other housemates, and another to share with a friend who currently lived by himself. I opted for the two-person share, but it's interesting to think what would have happened had I chosen the larger household, as I was a pain to be around at the time. My friend asked for $600 a month, but after I explained to him how much he needed me as a housemate and that I would "run the household", I was able to negotiate him down to $500, everything included. He is an oil rig worker, so he is frequently away; I told him I would pay the bills, look after the house, etc. I wanted to test run what it would be like to own my own home, so I thought this was a great opportunity. I also came up with the idea of paying all my bills upfront, so whatever money I had leftover could be spent with peace of mind. This resulted in me giving him $2,000 for the damage deposit and three months' rent. The lease was to begin in September, but as I was so eager to experience "freedom" from my parents, he said I could move in in August. I was extremely excited, and the day after I paid him and signed the lease, I began moving out.

I moved all my stuff to his place in a matter of three days, which took everyone by surprise as they were expecting me to move out in

September. I couldn't leave my parents' place fast enough, as I felt "small" around them – like a kid living at home. I wanted to feel like a man, because I was convinced that I was the man that would change the world, and to do that I would need a space of my own.

While I was in the process of moving out, my parents went to the United States for a shopping weekend. It was my job to look after our pets, and I ultimately failed them – I neglected to feed and water my dog one day. My mom was livid when she came home. She texted me, "I hope you have a conscience." I felt terrible, but I blamed it on six hours of sleep and being busy. "Busy thinking. Busy scheming. Busy listening. Busy planning and busy trying to make this world better." My mother was still not impressed and sent me two photos of my dog looking sad to try and guilt me. It worked to some degree, but I was so absorbed with the move, I continued unpacking and working on the house as if nothing had happened.

I had visited my grandparents during my move to the new house, and they offered to give me some housewarming gifts. My grandpa has a lot of cool stuff at his house, and I saw a box of vintage beer glasses that I just had to have. He invited me to take a few, but I wanted the whole box – I was going to make a display for them in the new garage. He agreed to let me take the entire box, but I just completely forgot about them as I was so easily distracted during my mania.

I remember my grandpa showing me a family history project he was working on in his office. I wrote some words of encouragement for him: "WHY CAN'T DALE BE AN AUTHOR? AND WHY CAN'T JASON BE A ROCKSTAR, A NOVELIST AND AN AUTHOR?" Because I couldn't pick *one* thing I wanted to be, I picked *all* things.

My excitement for a new westside home continued to grow after I left my grandparents' place. My parents' northside place seemed to be a symbol of who I had been, and the westside seemed like a new world – a free world. As I said to myself in an audio journal, "I need to get out of the old space. There are too many 'fuck off' moments at home. Screw the small thinkers." I thought my parents were the small thinkers; in reality, they were just trying to keep me grounded, but I was having none of it.

One morning at the new place I woke up hungry. We had cereal, but no milk, and it was a weekday so my nearest neighbour, Derrick, wasn't home. I decided I didn't want to go to the store, so I looked around the neighbourhood, cereal bowl in hand, at which houses still had cars parked out front. Surely not everyone in the neighbourhood was at work, I thought. The house across the street had an SUV parked out front, so I thought I would knock on the door and see if they could spare some milk – because, I remembered, in Tanzania everyone in the community is treated like family. A woman with a child on her hip answered the door, and I explained to her how I had just moved in and hadn't gone grocery shopping. I asked her if she could spare some milk. Luckily, she was a very nice woman, and happily agreed. She came out to the porch with a glass of milk and said I could keep the cup. I thanked her, and then made a little speech about how I was going to change the neighbourhood. The house I was staying in was known on the block for being the Party House. Derrick described walking out one morning to discover his child almost stepping in vomit on his front lawn from a party guest the night before. The woman I was speaking with also voiced her concerns when I told her I was at number 426, as the music was regularly too loud, and it disrupted her children's sleep.

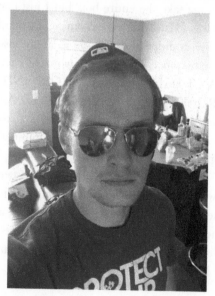

I vowed to both neighbours that a "new sheriff" was in town and that I would fix my housemate's disrespectful ways. I told them how I had learned abroad that community is the most important thing, and that there should be a sacred bond between you and your neighbours. The woman was happy with this, and I cheerfully went back to my new home, giddy at the thoughts in my head about how I would change this community for the better.

In addition to improving my new community, I was also trying to improve my new house. My ideas for improvements were endless. I was going to finish the unfinished garage and unfinished basement, and even renovate the kitchen. I wanted the house to be mine in a sense. I was rolling with these ideas, and I even thought I could turn it into a business – "Home Improvements" would be me and my housemate renovating homes super-fast. It was one of many business ideas I had, and it was just that, an idea. Nothing came out of this, other than me procrastinating unpacking my belongings.

Three Big Ideas

On 16 August, about two days after I had moved out, I recorded, "I feel like I'm not sleeping enough. I feel flu sick. It's been a process overload lately." But I shook off these concerns with one of my favourite sayings at the time: "The definition of good work is more work!" And said how it was my role in this world to "bring the Third World into the First World." I went on to come up with three big ideas.

The first was an app called "Freebies" – a mapping program providing the locations of stuff people want to give away. The second idea was "Textbooks Abroad". I have always been frustrated with how our university will give students 25 cents for secondhand $200 textbooks. In fairness, they have an overflow of stock, and publishers regularly update textbooks, making the old editions obsolete. My solution to this was to gather up old textbooks and send them to Tanzania. I didn't bother considering how I would cover the costs of shipping and handling. Lastly, I had the idea of gathering up free pianos and then finding homes for them. I got the idea from a Facebook advert for a free piano I was interested in. I've never played the piano, but I thought having one at the new house would be cool. Unfortunately, I was too late to claim it, and the owner said she destroyed it as a result. I was angry that such a fine instrument would go to waste, hence the rehoming idea. Again, how I would move these pianos and where I would store them went unconsidered. Thinking up these ideas redirected my focus away from how ill I was feeling, which is how my brain worked during this period. One thought would jump to another and then another and then another.

Becoming Prime Minister

"A life worth living is worth recording," I said to myself on 17 August, quoting Tony Robbins, of course. I had woken up after a brief sleep to no breakfast again, as I had still neglected to go grocery shopping. I ordered a breakfast sandwich and coffee for pickup. It was early in the morning, and after I picked up my breakfast, I began yet another audio journal. "The sheep are coming awake [sic] for another day of dreaming," I said, thinking that I was a lion that ate sheep for breakfast. I was extremely confident in my abilities, and felt like a dominant being. I was quite arrogant, come to think of it. I went down the rabbit hole of communism to start this day's journal, and came up with the idea of "Communist Capitalism", where the government meets all a person's needs, but somehow a free market economy still operates. How this would work, I still don't know. I then said how I would be my city's Tim Ferriss, because "I'm restless and efficient as shit!" Commenting on why I thought I would be successful, I said, "I wake up early and go to bed late because I have more energy than anybody. Enjoy the morning and be superhuman! And re-think time."

I explained in the same audio journal how I could be a "positive con man" by playing tricks and manipulating "bad people," so I could be a real-life superhero. I was proud of my contentment and said to my imaginary haters, "Sorry for finding contentment, read a fucking book."

I thought I had tapped into superhuman abilities and that I could "recall any memory at any time". I was convinced I had a photographic memory. I told myself to "Keep the Tanzania/African mindset" that I had during the trip. "Think big and act big", I liked to say.

One of the more significant ideas I had was how it would be easy to become the Prime Minister. I said in that same audio journal, "There is a plan for me to become Prime Minister. Hell, that's a novel idea: *One Man's Path to Becoming Prime Minister*." This plan, in addition to all my other ideas, I was convinced would happen. Because "I create the reality," I said. "You'll make millions!" I said to my future self.

I concluded this audio journal entry saying, "Voice recordings work well because, wow, does this mind race." Throughout my audio journals, I can see myself analyzing some of the symptoms of my manic episode, such as the lack of sleep, racing thoughts and rapid speech. I was unaware that I was severely ill and in a manic episode. Instead, I thought I had tapped into superhuman resources that made me invincible.

I was so excited about everything in my life that I had to tell as many people who would listen, and I thought the best channel for reaching as many people as possible was through my email and social media accounts.

Email

About a week home from the trip, on 16 August, I sent my Education 1000 teacher mentor (the second one) an overwhelming email, describing my trip and future ambitions. It was extremely long and very scattered. I started with asking him if he would like to meet up for a coffee, and that I would share a few thoughts in the email. A few turned into a lot. I told him how I thought I had lined myself up with a facilitation position with the organization I had travelled with, which was definitely not true. I talked about how "easy and cheap" it would be to fly to the moon in 50 years – "Save up, because it'll be less than $100k," I told him. Where I came up with that number, I have no idea. Staying on the topic of space, I asked him if he wanted to colonize Mars, because that was happening too, and "ANYTHING, anything at all is possible." I mentioned how I was "rambling a bit" in the email, but continued to ramble on. I wrote that I was "getting fired up sharing these thoughts." I tried to conclude with, "My final thought (for now) is that I am so grateful our paths crossed," which would have been a nice way to end the email. But, actually, I wasn't finished rambling. I went on to say, "I feel it is my CALLING to help as many youth and as many people find that passion, that obsession AND let them know that ANYTHING is possible if you're passionate and committed enough. The WHY is so much more important than the HOW."

Today, I would challenge that premise, as any SMART goal has 'A for Attainable' as the third step, which is something I completely overlooked during my mania. I came up with lofty goals, made up reasons why they would matter, but never took significant steps to make them actionable objectives.

I finished off the email with a massively long sentence: "... arrive in Canada, move out, postpone school for a year, bartend at the top night club in town, get hired as a seasonal facilitator with the organization I travelled with, travel the world or maybe teach in China, find a niche as an international teacher, learn six languages, come back and revolutionize the provincial curriculum, share world-class teaching techniques, teach people how to teach OR career switch and become this generation's Roger Waters, political musician, finally saying what I truly want to say to the world in the form of an album/tour in addition to a dystopian, Orwellian novel. I'd love to share more if you're interested. Let me know!" I left him my phone number and also attached pictures and videos of the trip in a second email.

As expected, he never replied. I'd be impressed if he actually got through the entire email at all, as it is quite a long read at 1,300 words.

I sent another email three days later in the early hours to my friend from the Tanzania trip and "business partner", Quinn. In this email, I explained some of my wild business plans and ambitions. "I want to BE one of those BRILLIANT young 20-something millennials that literally shocks the world with their 'overnight' success. It all sounds crazy, but I mean crazy runs the world, and being the right amount of crazy will make you a ton of money."

This email illustrates that, after being home for about a week and a half, I was starting to acknowledge that I may be a little crazy, but I thought that that was a good thing. I thought I was anything but ill. I believed I was doing better than ever, and I wanted to start sharing with people how I got to this new level.

I asked Quinn if he would "join me in this idea of Monthly Mutual Mentorship (MMM)". I told him, "I will respectfully decline SOCIETY'S pleads [sic] to 'SLOW DOWN' because this much progress intimidates the common man. But Quinn and Jason are NOT common, and why would you want to be common anyway? The common are easily manipulated and unsatisfied. … Why can't we conquer the world with our brilliance? Who cares that we're 15 and 20? Guess what! Tony Robbins, Richard Branson, Bill Gates, Steve Jobs, Quinn and Jason ALL faced a TON of adversity and GREW from it to become SUPER Performers." My confidence was high, and my ideas were rolling.

I shared with Quinn a new obsession of mine. "Quinn, what if we created a micro group (5–8 people to start) that ARE the Super Performers in our World (i.e., you, me, my brilliant friends and yours) and created a monthly micro chat of excellence where we make a mini competition with each other to decide who can be the MOST successful (their own definition of success) in 30 days. Anyways, enough Wegner Rambling for now (it's 5:34am where I am, but I am loving this early morning Super Performer trend of 'winning the morning')."

This email to Quinn was the beginning of my new Facebook group "Master Minding", and I emailed the original members of the group next, outlining my ambitions and goals for the group.

Master Minding

The Master Minding email was sent to the 15 people I thought were the most efficient, effective and successful people in my life. I told them about the idea of a "small group on Facebook and email of Super Performers, that share/collaborate on BIG ideas, share meaningful/useful (on a daily micro- and lifelong macro-level) resources AND have a space to think, build ideas on, find new ideas and just collaborate with like-minded excellence, etc." This email was sent at 6:14am on 19 August, about 45 minutes after my email to Quinn. I told the group, "I will handle the mini membership process because too many people trying to Master Mind in such a small space will defeat the purpose." I had low expectations for the reception of this email: "My expectation is that four out of fifteen people will want to join, and that is okay." After the email, I got to work building the group page on Facebook and adding members.

I actually got some excellent responses – one friend said she was "excited to be a part of the group", and another said she loved it. These comments were encouraging, so I posted regularly. I began with, "Don't get on my case for me being me, because then we have a problem." The group eventually grew to about 40 people, and I wanted it to be this great collaboration page. In reality, it was just another manic journal. No one really posted, except me. Half the group saw most of the long and scrambled posts, but rarely "liked" them.

I shared some personal thoughts in the posts, and rationalized this by saying, "If you sweep too many things under the rug you'll trip and get a concussion and wow look, now you've got brain damage when all you had to do was speak and share." So, I shared a lot.

My good friend Scotty brilliantly posted a quote on the page from Emile Zola: "If I cannot overwhelm with my quality, I will overwhelm with my quantity." I was definitely being overwhelming. I mostly did shout-outs and introductions, but I also used the page to describe the big moments that occurred during the weeks leading to my hospitalization. I was actively trying to create big moments in my life, as I said in one post, "What if you pretended right now that you were writing your fascinating, future bestselling autobiography?" This post turned out to be a little ironic, given that I *am* writing a book about my experiences right now.

I wasn't too upset that the group never really took off, as I said, "If this Master Minding group dies and never becomes more than an online journal for myself to reflect on that's fine. I've already had many victories and breakthroughs the last few days, and this page and all of you silently reading these thoughts feels good and has seriously helped me out."

Most of my posts were "free posts", which is a term I came up with to describe a post that isn't edited and is just stream of consciousness writing – what comes to mind, write it down. I also implored members to "opt out" at any time, as I wanted no negativity in the group. The page aimed to be a space where members (mostly me) could share their thoughts that needed reaffirming in real-time and be shared with the most trusted and brilliant of friends. I told the group, "I have not been the Jason Wegner that everyone knew before the trip to Tanzania. I'm not going to be that version of myself anymore, because it's fake."

I was never apologetic for the content overload: "I'm not sorry for posting this much, for being at a level ten energy all day or for being myself!" I was convinced that I understood the brain, and wrote, "Understand the brain, and you unlock an abundant source of power." But this "power" was merely manic energy that was unsustainable and would eventually get me into trouble.

12

THE JUNGLE FIRING

After sending out emails, starting the Master Minding group and smoking some pot, I remembered I had a big shift at The Jungle that night, as there was a huge wedding being put on in the ballroom. It was one of my first shifts back since the trip. I had ambitious goals to transform The Jungle into the best bar on the westside of town, but it looked like nothing had changed in the three weeks I'd been away. I was disappointed and furious that nearly a month of potential progress had been lost. However, my boss Ron had actually done two significant things while I was gone: changed the draft beer system and got approval for liquor guns. I was oblivious to this, and it upset him that I came back with such a bad attitude. However, my mental health was such that I wasn't really affected by his displeasure. I was becoming obstinately manic.

The wedding night shift started at 4pm, and I was scheduled to stay until closing time. I was at a level ten of enthusiasm and, being the most experienced bartender on the staff that night, I felt like I was commander in chief. It was a busy affair after the ceremony and dinner. Lines were long, but we were pumping drinks out fast. It was an open bar, so we didn't have to worry about taking money, just serving the drinks. I was having a blast as I love to bartend, and not having to worry about money was awesome. I was flirting with women and having fun with all the customers. I thought my energy was contagious, as it seemed like people were drawn to my "off the wall" character. One lady was upsetting me, however, as she was blocking her cute friends from talking to me and was being sloppy with her alcohol. I thought she'd had too much to drink, so I cut her off. Doing this was a bad idea as she was a bridesmaid, and she immediately complained to the bride and groom. I didn't care though.

Because we were so busy, I came up with what I thought was a brilliant idea. My line would be highballs only, the middle line cans only and the third line cocktails only. My thinking was that this would be more efficient, but also most advantageous for me because quick highballs get big tips on a busy night. My co-workers agreed, and all the good traffic was headed my way. Of course, we had our tip jars out, I made sure of that, but there was some confusion as there was also a "host" tip jar. This jar was meant to be a cash donation to the bride and groom to help cover liquor costs. Our jars had no sign on them, and people were confused as to which jar was for which purpose. The groom saw that I was making the most drinks and the most tips, so he put the host jar beside my overflowing tip jar. This upset me because my tips went down as a result. I moved the host jar back to the middle, and told the other bartenders to keep pushing it to the middle of the bar if it got moved again. This caused a problem between the groom and me, and he let my boss Ron know it.

Ron came over to me and said I needed to take a break. We went outside for a talk; he lit up a smoke, and I asked for one. I told him I had started smoking in Africa, and he agreed to give me one. He was quite upset with my behaviour, and let me know it. He cited me cutting off and arguing with a bridesmaid, and then accused me of getting people to put money in my tip jar, thinking it was the host tip jar. He said I had to talk to the owner, Terri, and explain what was going on, because the groom wanted me off the shift.

I called Terri, and she asked me how much I thought I was going to make in tips that night, as nobody at The Jungle had ever walked out with more than a couple of hundred dollars in one night. I told her I expected to make $400, and that I shouldn't be punished for being good at my job. I explained my side of the story, and also how I was tired from moving and still readjusting to North America. I don't think I really apologized for any of my behaviours, I just tried to rationalize them. We talked some more, and I thought everything was okay, and I would be able to go back to work. She briefly spoke with Ron, and Ron said I had to leave. He said the groom was too upset, so I had to go. They said we would figure this all out at a later date.

I took my tips, tipped out my co-workers handsomely and walked out the back door, avoiding the groom. I got in my truck and drove away from the bar pretty upset, and began an audio journal that would last 74 minutes.

I was at a level ten in anger and was pretty much shouting into my phone during this recording. I was resolved to going home, getting stoned and forgetting about everything. I said, "Fuck The Jungle, it's part of the past… I put people first and they still sent me home," which was a comment on how I thought I was giving excellent service to the party. I was mad that the groom "tattled" on me to my boss, but in hindsight, what groom wouldn't? But I didn't have such rational thoughts at the time. I thought, "Maybe I should fuck off from North America." And then reminded myself, "I control everything", and followed that up with the elitist thought: "I'm like a God. Do I think I'm a God? No." As I was saying this, I almost drove into oncoming traffic – luckily, I didn't crash. The recording of my angry thoughts continued.

"Fuck the system. Was I an asshole tonight? Yeah. But nobody understands. I'm not a bad guy." At this thought, I was starting to get a bit teary, which was a display of my drastic mood swings, another symptom of bipolar disorder. I went on to say I was "ready to quit at any time. I don't want to be somewhere where I can't be myself, can't be unchained and am told to slow down." By this point, I was parked outside my house; if I was still at the bar, I might have gotten into a fight, as I "wanted to punch the groom in the face!" But I then told myself, "Calm the fuck down." I questioned my whole life: "Why don't I live a normal life that is less stressful and less focussed on massive goals?" Then immediately said, "Naw, FUCK THAT!"

I went on a rant, saying I was "in the management game. In the 'change the world' game. I can get on anyone's radar." I spoke about my tenacity as I described myself as a "fuck you" kind of guy:

"Obstructing progress? Well fuck you, let's get in the ring!" And back to The Jungle train of thought, I said, "I could do the manager's job so much better." Winded from speaking for so long, I even said, "It's so hard to shut the fuck up!"

I then got serious and reflected on how "I've been so rattled in North America because I haven't had the chance to listen." This thought definitely had some truth to it, as I spent a lot of time talking and almost no time listening. I swung back to anger pretty quickly with, "North America is fucking stupid." I was mad at the government and mad at the whole world. I asked, "What would Tony Robbins do? What would his advice be?" Then I thought, "What would Roger Waters do?" I decided that I still wanted to "slap that groom silly, as he was the asshole, not me." I jumped back to Tanzania: "I figured it out in Tanzania. I have a vision. I am bold, intimidating and cocky, but apparently, enthusiasm is off-putting." I got sad again: "I've been through adversity. I've been told to stop being myself because I am too intense, and that hurts." I picked myself up quickly, however, "I'm crazy and crazy runs the world." I explained how I had no regrets and how "I would do this day the same all over again." I started to close off, saying, "Enough talking. I've been up for a really long time." But I wasn't finished – I still had another 47 minutes' worth of thoughts to get off my chest.

"Moving out was the tipping point, because I now have a space where I can be me." Then, jumping to another thought, I asked the world, "Will somebody teach me how to shut the hell up?" I got emotional again, "I have the power to change the world. I'm in the youth empowerment game and the business building game. Adults don't think big enough." I was now fired up, "I can outperform greatness. I am superhuman. ... I don't want financial abundance. I want total financial abundance."

I tried to make this idea of total financial abundance real with the big scheme of launching my corporation, Wegner Ways Incorporated (WWInc.). I said that "WWInc. will have private schools, bars, movies, TV shows, novels, articles, technology, luxury airline services and, above all, music." With these big ideas, I thought, "I need to get out of town because I am too intense. I might screw off to San Francisco and build my empire there." I expressed the urgency of these ideas: "I don't have time to waste. I don't have time for little people. I have all the ideas and all the energy, and I can come up with great ideas on no food." I also mentioned how "people think I am crazy," but that was never really of great concern to me.

I was getting exhausted, as I had been rambling for almost an hour after a seven-hour shift on a day that had begun at 5am with the emails. I ended on inspiration: "I am a real-world superhero. I can be anything I want to be, even a painter! Any day is a good day. Tony Robbins will endorse me one day, and I will work for him. Hell, I'm gonna buy a country one day and run it! I am a rational, brilliant human."

Finally, at 1am, I got out of my truck and walked to the backyard to smoke some pot and go to bed. I thought all was good at The Jungle and that this night would blow over, but I was wrong.

A few days later, my boss Ron had me call him and the owner to discuss the wedding shift. They informed me that there had been a major complaint, and it looked awful for the business. They said they would have to let me go. I didn't really care, however, and told them that I was okay and that I was going to quit anyway because I had bigger plans to execute and work on.

After the phone call, Terri emailed me, "You definitely sounded very positive, passionate and visionary about your future, and I think that's great. ... I'd be remiss if I didn't reach out to you also and let you know that if you are having difficulty with the outcome of this resolution, or if you're shouldering any other concerning matters that there are campus services available." She included, at the bottom of the email, a link to the university's counselling services. She was obviously concerned about my well being, as were a lot of people; but I didn't understand everybody's problem with me. I was on top of the world. I didn't care that I had just been fired from a job I loved. I was going to change the world. I decided that, as I wasn't working at The Jungle anymore and only getting minimal shifts at the catering company, I would volunteer.

13

20 AUGUST

I was very optimistic after being sent home from The Jungle, and was even celebrating being sent home, as documented in a Snapchat video I made while on a morning walk around 6am (which is something I would start doing regularly). I said I was "standing up for what I believe in," which I guess suggests I still thought I was in the right about the night before.

Good Intentions

I wasn't hungry, so I thought I would try to volunteer at the middle school where my mom was working. They were doing renovations and had said they could use some volunteers. I drove down to the school and parked across the street in front of somebody's house. Before going to volunteer, I became distracted by my phone and ended up scrolling for nearly an hour. Then, my old coach Trevor called me. He had sent me a text a few days earlier commenting on my Master Minding posts: "You may want to consider writing everything out clearly and then re-reading it a day later before posting it. Good energy, though!" I replied that I didn't have the time or patience to wait a day before every post, but thanked him anyway. In the phone call, I remember him being concerned about my stream of consciousness writing, and was worried that I hadn't readjusted to North America yet. We talked (well, I talked) for about an hour, and I did my best to reassure him that I was fine and that I had just taken my life to another level of peak performance. I truly believed that there was nothing wrong with me, but I'm sure I didn't put Trevor at ease.

After the phone call, I was audio journaling when the owner of the house I was parked in front of came out. She asked, "What the heck are you doing?" I reassured her that I was here to volunteer at the school, but had just been caught up in some very important business dealings. I then told the owner of the house about my volunteer app idea called "Minga". The app would be like an Uber app, but for volunteers, I said. Basically, it would allow people to log in and be volunteers for however long they wanted and would get other users to drop pin locations to where they needed help. I told her how I thought it would be great for seniors who need help with random tasks, such as mowing their lawn or organizing their garage. *Minga* is a word I learned in Ecuador – it is what locals shout out to their community members when they need help with a task. I asked the lady if she thought the app was a good idea, and she said it was a "great idea". We instantly became friends, and I got her contact information and told her that the app would go live in September.

The app would, of course, not be launched in September, but I still don't think it's an entirely bad idea. If there are any readers out there that want to steal the idea and make it a reality, by all means, make it happen. I have zero experience of app development, and I am really not much of a computers guy.

I finally walked over to the school to start volunteering, oblivious to what time it was. I had, in fact, been parked outside the school for nearly three hours. By the time I reached the school they were already done for the day, as it was hot and they had started early in the morning. I was upset at this North American work schedule because, in Africa, the locals worked on their school building project from sunrise to sundown. Disgusted at the laziness of the North Americans, I headed home.

When I got home, I read a short email my friend Tom had sent me. He said he was really liking the Master Minding group idea, so I enthusiastically wrote a long reply. In it, I said, "I know this has been a massive content overload with the latest posts, but I am consciously doing this. My only aim is to make this an AWESOME space we can ALL use (or not use) whenever." I then said, "You have the ability to shut me up any time you like," which was probably the biggest lie I told throughout my entire manic episode, as it was nearly impossible to shut me up. I closed with, "I'm not apologizing for 'being at a ten' or 'being too enthusiastic' because that's garbage. Don't like it? Then turn me off. GET USED TO IT, SOCIETY!" Tom didn't respond to this, which I don't blame him for. He had merely given me a little support, and I turned it into a shouty email all about myself.

I was starting to feel hungry as I hadn't eaten all day and it was nearly 5pm. A few days earlier, I had run into my old Grade 6 teacher, and he had agreed to have coffee with me at 7pm, so I figured I ought to get something to eat before meeting him. I grabbed my backpack, which I had basically made as a "run away from home" bag that I called the "Certainty Pack". It had everything you would need if you ever ran away or found yourself not wanting to go home: a toothbrush, fresh underwear, sunscreen, bug screen, deodorant, a towel, water, journals and, of course, marijuana. So, with my backpack in hand, I drove to a restaurant near the place we were meeting for coffee, and came up with my next big idea.

The Napkin

Feeling particularly famished, but also financially responsible, I asked the bartender what the special was. It was a steak sandwich, and I saw that as a sign that the universe was smiling at me because it was my favourite meal. I ordered it with a side of sweet potato fries and a Coke. While waiting for my food, I found my mind racing. I had left my "Certainty Pack" in my truck, but I always had a pen with me. With no paper around, I began writing on a nearby napkin. Here, I would describe, in great detail, the bar I would create.

I wrote, "James is my main man", as I thought I would go into business with my old bartending mentor. I then listed all the potential employees – mostly former co-workers of mine who were phenomenal at their job – and wrote that I would focus on "building a team". I wrote that I would "poach the best" from other bars and restaurants and create the ultimate working environment. I would "facilitate awesomeness". I might call it "BJ's Sports Bar" – B for beer and J for joints; the sexual innuendo never dawned on me! There would be affordable drinks with "transparent tipping", which meant that the bar managers would never be tipped out by servers, as this was something that enraged me when I worked at Duncan's Pub. I wrote down and drew the "Fast Lane Bar Service" for the quick drinks, and the "Specialty Lane" for cocktails and specialty drinks. I was basically recreating what I had thought was a brilliant idea the night before at The Jungle. I wrote, "I've always wanted my own bar," so all my ideas on the napkin were what I thought would make the ultimate bar. Our slogan would be "Bud, Buds and Bud", meaning "Budweiser, Buddies, and Marijuana Bud". I thought it was clever at the time. "THINK BIG ACHIEVE BIG."

I wrote I would "rethink the outdated hiring process" and somehow improve it. I described what kind of boss I'd be: I would perform "sneaky tests on staff, watch them all the time [and] invoke FEAR." I guess it would be my place to be a mini dictator, which I thought would lead to the ideal working environment. At this point, I did question what I was doing, and wrote, "Why do we take notes?" and responded with, "My biggest fear is that I'll forget." I wanted to capture this moment in time, so I also wrote down what I was eating, and then got lost in another train of thought.

About 45 minutes into writing on this single napkin, I wrote, "I'm not in the teaching, business or bartending game. I'M IN THE EMPIRE GAME... I can literally live as an abundant overnight 20-year-old Tycoon within weeks! WHAT THE HELL AM I WAITING FOR!?" I described how my business would fund my charity People First, and how I would have Prime Minister Trudeau backing me because of my connection to him. I also listed three former professors of mine who I was sure would jump on board. I discussed the urgency of everything as I wrote, "Live the life you wanna live now, seriously act now before fear or THE SOCIETY BRINGS YOU DOWN." I continued to write how this would be the best bar ever, and how I would make sure I "hooked my people up in more ways than they expected". I would "make sure ALL THEIR needs were met, i.e., health, shelter, medical (products and education on weed), resources, etc.".

I planned a backroom "legit Psychedelic Experience Package", where the bar would give you psychedelic drugs and then take you on a spiritual journey. I was definitely not thinking of the legalities of supplying illicit drugs at my bar, but I thought it was a cool idea. I also came up with another app called "Biz Builders", where "we do all the math" in your prospective business venture. I noted that this would be an app "that will make me money". Obviously, calculating all the factors and numbers a business needs to run a successful operation would be very difficult to cram into an app, but if any readers want to steal that app idea too, by all means, go for it.

I wrote that I had to "literally make it happen and make it happen fast. It's not hard. WHEN WOULD NOW BE A GOOD TIME?" Now, sitting at the bar of a busy restaurant and scribbling like a madman onto a napkin for an hour, obviously attracted some attention

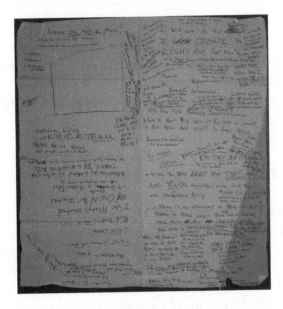

and I noticed this when I was finished. After I had paid my bill, I wrote on a second napkin "Hey you! Remember that guy sitting on that chair writing on that napkin? Give him five years and then Google 'Jason Wegner napkin'. Get in touch with me, it'll be easy, and I'd love to meet you because this note found you for a reason. Cheers!" And as I walked out with my brilliant napkin in hand, I saw the man who was sitting next to me grab the second napkin. I smiled and walked out the door.

I still had a few minutes to kill before meeting my old teacher, so I went and sat in the field that overlooked a local high school. I sat there, belly and heart full with immense contentment. I dreamed of my future high school classroom, teaching novels and reading stories to teenagers. I then thought of all my other big plans. "A bright future indeed," I thought to myself. Aware of the time, I calmly rose from the ground and moseyed on over to the coffee shop where I could feel my excitement building, as I couldn't wait to fill Mr B, my sixth-grade teacher, in on all the wonderful things going on in my life.

Mr B

While Mr B grabbed us coffee, I got us a seat out on the patio and sneakily began recording, as I thought this conversation might have the potential to make it onto the Wegner Ways Podcast one day. I didn't ask for permission from Mr B, which I should have, but I didn't really care. To start, I warned Mr B, "I am in the business of speed," and that he should brace himself. I then told him how I had "unlimited resources" was "gonna revolutionize the school curriculum." He knew of Tim Ferriss, so I said, "*4-Hour Workweek*? What? Are you lazy? How about the '2-Hour Workweek'!?" I asked him questions, but was speaking so fast he never had a chance to reply. I told him I wanted to be a "master at listening", which was unintentionally ironic and obviously something I never strived towards in my mania. I told him all about how I had "learned to scheme" and come up with big ideas. "I wanna be a villain for the bad guys", so like an anti-hero. After 29 minutes of me talking, I asked him a question, but then rambled on for another ten minutes. I was continually changing topics, yet told him, "Losing the train of thought is how the brain works," which is how the *manic* brain works. I wouldn't even give him ten seconds to think of a question when he asked for a moment to think. I was on a high like no other.

I commented on his body language in mid-sentence, like how he was seated, where his arms were placed, etc.; he said, "How are you engaged in conversation, but so hyper-aware of someone else's body language?"

I replied, "That's just how my brain works." And that was true – the manic brain is hyper-aware of everything; it is always thinking, and thinking fast.

I was telling Mr B about all of my ideas and the "seven businesses I created" the night before, when I casually mentioned that I had been fired from work. My firing intrigued Mr B, and he wanted to know the story. I replied, "People are living in a daydream," and then went down a completely different rabbit hole. Listening back to this recording to write this book was hard at times, because I genuinely do sound insane. It's hard to listen to your voice making random noise and rambling about nothing to someone you look up to.

After continuing to ramble and not answering Mr B's question about The Jungle, I said, "I'm rare. I'm a super learner... We have a Canadian Tony Robbins in our backyard," referring to myself, which was quite delusional. At 20, I was nowhere near the stature of the megastar that is Tony Robbins, but I sure thought I was on his level. Twenty-five minutes after Mr B asked the question about me getting fired, I circled back to it and asked him, "How do you define good work?" I, of course, didn't let him answer the question, and told him how I had "discovered myself in Tanzania, discovered that I needed to reinvent myself." Aware of my thinking, I said, "We're all over the place, but that is how my mind works... I may not have all the secrets in the world, but I have all the questions, and questions get answers." Well, they get answers if you let other people speak, which is something I had trouble with.

Jumping to career aspirations, I said, "If I can't speak freely as a teacher, then I'll become a professor and say whatever the hell I want."

At this, Mr B finally got a word in and said, "Jason, I am enthralled by your speaking."

I got emotional and said, "I'm doing everything so fast because I am scared like hell that I'm not going to follow through," which was a real fear at the time. I spoke about my mental health, "Call me crazy … maybe I'm insane, or maybe I'm on the same wavelength as all of these brilliant super performers because I actually listened to them!" I was the former, not the latter in this case. I thought I was brilliant, but in reality, I was severely mentally ill. Because I thought I was such a "super performer", I said to Mr B, "I could write a book about my life right now!" I thought my story of overcoming adversity and getting on this new level of super performance would be worth writing about. A book would indeed be written (and you are reading it right now), but it would, of course, be drastically different to what I imagined during my mania.

We eventually got to the topic of reverse culture shock, which I told Mr B, "is a thing, big time." I told him how, when I came home from Tanzania, "I couldn't stop thinking."

Concerned, Mr B asked, "How are you dealing with that right now?"

I replied, "By scheming, audio journaling, writing thoughts down, and talking to my network of people, because it is fricking hard."

He then asked, "Do you find that you have individuals in your life that you feel, if you were to share that with them, they would crush it?"

To this, I gave an extensive reply. "100 per cent. That's why I moved across town. Because my dad lost his job," which was true. "My mom has to go back to work a few days earlier and the school isn't finished being renovated and they're both stressed out in their own life. And my dog is sick, and my great grandfather is sick as well. Like everything is happening all at once again." Angered, I continued, "I was like, fuck this. I was so mad because I thought it was so unfair." This thought bridged to a memory about returning from Arizona the previous summer. "Last year, Dad picked me up in my truck at the airport and didn't even ask how my trip to Arizona was. I told my grandparents how hurtful that was. After I had done all this advanced facilitator training, he asked first, 'How was the weather?' And then told me that he lost his job and has to borrow my vehicle for a while. Then I didn't get to talk at all about my Arizona experience, which I was really proud of because I was one of out of thousands of kids to be invited to learn there. It was a Tony Robbins, life-changing experience I went through, and my dad crushed that experience. He didn't even realize it. And it wasn't even fair to be mad at him because he was just being himself. I fell into the trap of learning all these great things and world-changing ideas in Arizona and did nothing with them. I learned lots but didn't execute any of it. Talk is nice, but walking is living." This was one of the main reasons why I was so driven to make a change when I got home from Tanzania. I didn't want to come home and do nothing with all that I had learned.

I was quite emotional after this speech, and Mr B comforted me saying, "You're a good man Jason, and don't forget that or beat yourself up. I'm sorry you had to go through that with your dad."

I switched to optimism after the long speech about me and my dad. "What if I lived my life pretending, I had to write a book about it when I'm 95? Maybe an anthology!" Staying with the optimism, I told him about my napkin idea. After that, I said, in the third person, "Jason's mind is everywhere all at once! Don't be a master in minor things. Be an expert in all things!" I also mentioned that I would "destroy the idea of the Third World".

Mr B said, "I really have to go." To finally wrap up the long conversation that was nearing the two-hour mark, I got serious.

"My definition of success is determined by how many people I impact."

To this, Mr B replied, "Are you okay about who you are when you look in the mirror at night when no one else is around?"

I answered with an emphatic yes, as I genuinely was confident in my abilities and happy with myself during this period. While I did have some lows during my manic episode where I would feel quite sad, I had so many highs that they made me forget about feeling down.

I walked Mr B to his car and thanked him for meeting with me, and said we should do it again soon. I also casually mentioned that I had recorded the entire conversation and said I had already sent him a copy of it. He said, "You should really ask my permission if you're going to record," but I reassured him that it was just for him and me and that I wouldn't share it with anybody. I said it was for help with the memory. I asked him what the difference was between recalling a memory in your head versus listening to the memory word for word. We said goodbye, and he drove off to be with his family, who were probably wondering where he was!

Late-night Reflection

After speaking with Mr B, I did some journaling on my phone late into the night. I started the journal entry by quoting Mr B: "Even giants go to bed, Jason." I began to rattle off some thoughts, "I need to help teachers discover their brilliance," and said my writings would "be on thousands of teachers' phones one day". Energetic at this thought, I wrote, "Wegner has become unchained!!! I am unleashed. I am Me, AND I LOVE IT! And I'm still crazy. I feel like I have finally torn down THE WALL, which I created and has been working against me since day one. Well, I'm tired of walls." Then, trying to humble myself, I wrote, "It's not that I know everything... I actually feel like I know nothing. But at least I know how to ask a question... I'm done apologizing for being too... enthusiastic, loud, fast, shady, fat, analytical, late, curious, nosy, smelly, ugly, smart and myself. Be the bird that spreads the good word because the bird is the word. Confused yet? Good. Stay Curious." I then commented that I was "extremely tired" but followed that up by saying I need to "re-think sleeping and eating". And with that thought, I finished journaling for the night and drifted off to sleep at the reasonable hour of 3:30am. It had been a long, eventful day, but the following day would be even more interesting.

14

SMALL TOWN, USA

I made the decision, on a whim, to travel to the States for the day to pick up a $2,000 stereo that was waiting for me in a shipping business in a small border town about 90 minutes away from my city. The stereo, which had come all the way from Denmark, was supposedly the "best stereo in the world", according to Quinn. In addition to the stereo, I also went online shopping and bought a pair of sunglasses that played music through your skull not ears (they didn't work very well) and a brand new $1,200 computer, which was also supposedly "the best in the world" according to Quinn. I was into technology for sure, but this spending was a prime example of the Manic Man on full tilt. One of the risks of being in a manic episode is fiscal irresponsibility, and I was definitely displaying that. I didn't really need a new computer, especially one I had never seen in person, and I certainly didn't need a fancy new stereo.

This last-minute decision to travel to the States was very out of character − I am usually a very organized and plan-ahead kind of person. I was so unprepared that I even forgot my passport. I had a picture of my passport on my phone and, apparently, this was good enough for the American border security guard, as she let me cross no problem. On my way back into Canada, border security was shocked that the Americans had let me through, but I had a lot of luck that day.

I was enthralled to be in another country again, and at how quaint and straightforward this little border town was. When I walked into the shipping business, I was mostly focussed on the potential of the place. It was a bit dingy, but all I could think about was all the excellent global and American products you can't get in Canada. Surely, people would want a service that could access these. While the woman working the counter cashed me out, a boy, maybe 12 years old, went and got my package. I was impressed with his work ethic and saw a tip jar on the counter.

"Do the tips go to him?" I asked the woman.

"They sure do. This is my son," she replied. I gave him a $5 Canadian bill, picked up my stereo and headed to my truck. I looked at my new stereo, with its unique and futuristic cone design and decided I couldn't wait the two hours to get home to see how it sounded. So, I unboxed the stereo at my truck, found an electrical point outside the shipping business and connected my phone to the stereo. The boy came out to see what I was doing. I told him how he was about to see "the world's greatest stereo" on display. I played a Pink Floyd song at full volume, and watched his amazement at how loud and how far the sound went. I asked him what his favourite band was. He said he really liked Twenty One Pilots, who I also like. I played him their hit songs and struck up a conversation with him. I asked him what subjects he liked in school and if he liked to read books. He said school was "alright", that he liked gym class and didn't read much outside of school. I quizzed him and asked if Africa was a country or a continent. He said Africa was a country. I was disappointed at this, and went on a rant about how American education is too isolationist and needs to teach more about the rest of the world. I told him I was a big business guy from Canada, and that I was going to revolutionize the curriculum in Canada and then North America. The kid found me interesting, and I liked the kid.

I missed kids, to be honest. I had been surrounded by them in Tanzania – by teenagers as fellow participants and the local elementary-school children. In Tanzania, kids are raised by the community – kids are everybody's kids. It was perfectly normal during the trip to play or talk with a *watoto* (child) because there was supervision everywhere. I missed that, and I treated this exchange the same way I did any exchange in Tanzania. I told the boy I'd love to keep in contact and teach him more about the world. I didn't have any paper on me because I, thankfully, had left my "Certainty Pack" (with its marijuana) at home, so I wrote my contact information on a piece of cardboard and told him to Skype me between 11:30am and 2:30pm the next day. I also told him to read *Shoe Dog* by Phil Knight, the story of Nike, which I was listening to on Audible at the time. I drove away happy that I had made a new friend, and that I had seen a spark of curiosity in a child. I felt like I had made a real connection with that kid and that I would be able to change his life by staying in contact and teaching him the "Wegner Ways" of life. I was quite excited as I drove away. As I had no responsibilities for the rest of the day, I decided to drive around and discover more of what the border town had to offer.

The Field

I found a dusty road that led to a dead-end in an open field, and decided to park there and soak up the day. Excited about the excellent day I was having, I started a Snapchat video that would be accessible to all my friends and followers. I began with, "I'm on Tanzania Time." I then told everyone watching that, "I understand the brain. If you don't like the new me, then *kwaheri* (goodbye)." I then talked about my trip to small-town USA, and how I came up with a new business idea: "... sell from my garage, stuff from the USA you'll wanna buy. It's untapped potential and gonna be huge!" In the background of the video, I was playing "Small Town" by John Mellencamp. I implored my viewers that if they wanted the small-town USA experience, all they would have to do is ask me. I told them, "I live in abundance," and, "It's okay to be f-ing crazy. I am crazy." I spoke of my future: "I'm gonna be rich and make people rich." As I was recording this, I was lying on the back of my truck with the camera pointed at me. I told the invisible crowd, "You can live any way you want, NOW!" I told them to watch out for me because I "came up with the big one, like Apple, Nike, Google, Amazon, etc. I am unleashed!" I ended the video with, "I am done asking questions. Well, actually, I'm never done asking questions, but I am more than ever, ready to find more answers."

With that video to all my followers and friends over, I started a new one to send to just a few friends. It was another rant, this time about how "America is freedom". I demonstrated this freedom by videoing myself defecating in the middle of the field I was parked at, wiping myself with a towel and leaving it there "for the wild". It was a gross action and one I'm obviously not proud of – at the time I thought it was funny and making a point.

Big Ideas

After relieving myself in the field, I started journaling in my phone about the "big one". I wrote, "I need help starting a business asap." I wrote that this big business idea would "branch every sister business and fuel the charities from day one. I will use my 'overthinking'/ stressing over nothing behaviours to my entrepreneurial advantage." I was going to call the big business "Holistic Solutions or a name from a foreign language, i.e., Swahili, Spanish, etc." I then stated the primary goal of the business was to be, "A Professional Consulting service for small business owners in town and area, i.e., micro-efficiencies saving money, making fast ground-breaking solutions that happen NOW! What's wrong with your business? Need easy, fast, actionable advice?" Holistic Solutions would use "world-class ground-breaking 2017 solutions. Old solutions, new solutions, ALL THE SOLUTIONS!" I mentioned how I wanted to "be my own boss" and have the ability to "make money whenever I FEEL like it, and also while I am SLEEPING." This business would be "A ONE-STOP SHOP" and "a place where our team (my people) will, from a holistic and pragmatic framework, give you ACTIONABLE advice/ consultation in yes, as little as an hour." We would "charge based on the job". There would also be a place in the business where I could "give massive career advice... ALL THE ADVICE!!!" I spun the slogan, "Want FAST, EFFICIENT SOLUTIONS NOW? Well, our team of highly intelligent, efficient, young people will give you solutions within hours AND give you actionable plans that YOU can start ACTING upon easily after one consultation." I then asked the most critical question about this business idea, "Why would anyone want to take advice from me?" But left it unanswered, and jumped to other thoughts.

The next significant thought I had was how "I could literally buy a plane ticket and teach English abroad at any moment." I wrote how I could "start a micro tutoring service/reading workshop" and teach people how to speed read. "Wanna take your grades to the NEXT LEVEL? ... What if I could increase your reading speed and retention within a one-hour lesson?" I continued speaking to imaginary clients, "I'm no witch doctor, I just get results." When looking back at this journal, I realized that I had stolen this idea from Tim Ferriss, who ran this exact kind of workshop for his fellow students at Princeton. Ferriss is much more of an authority on super learner techniques than I am, but it was merely another one of my delusions that I could run such a workshop.

I also wrote, "YOU CAN GET PAID STARTING ON MONDAY BY JUST BEING EXCELLENT AT BEING YOU AND FIGURING OUT HOW TO MONETIZE YOUR AWESOMENESS." Basically, I believed that I was my greatest resource and asset. I ended this journal by telling myself to "... be an expert negotiator, teacher, and businessman — an expert in all. You live in abundance. Go out and give."

After Snapchatting and journaling for nearly two hours, I drove back to the centre of the town. I was starting to feel hungry as I hadn't eaten much all day, so I pulled into the local convenience store that was connected to a bar. As I was pulling up, the boy from the shipping company pulled up with his mom and dad. I was excited to see my new friend again and asked him if he would show me around the store and pick out the best thing to eat. He said the sandwiches are tasty, so I paid for one and then grabbed a seat in the empty bar, and he followed. I missed having lunch with kids like when I was in Africa, and I had mostly been eating alone since moving out of my parents' place. I began telling the boy more about my trip to Africa and also about my trip to Ecuador. I showed him some pictures and told him some stories, like the time I ate a live grub (insect) in Ecuador. He was captivated. I began telling him about my business plans, and how even the empty bar we were in could be part of my business. I was excited at the idea of a border-town bar. America can offer some things that Canada can't, and the ideas were rolling through my head. The boy said his uncle ran the bar, and I asked him to go get him because I had big ideas. I shared some of them with the uncle, and he humoured me. I mostly just asked questions and told him how much I loved the small town.

After I finished the sandwich, I got the uncle to sell me a beer, even though I was underage in the States. I took it outside to where a few regulars were sitting on the patio. For the most part, these strangers were friendly. I entered the conversation saying I was a big businessman in Canada, or that I was starting out anyways, and that I had big ideas for the town. One man, Rod, said his favourite thing in the world was seeing Canadians hit home runs out of Canada and into America, as there is a baseball field that backs onto the border in Canada. He said he loves baseball and that it makes him feel connected to his neighbours. I said I loved this too, and that I had other ideas to make the Canadian and American sides more connected. "Why can't a Canadian come down for a day and really experience what small-town USA is all about?" I asked. I then went on a tangent talking about US politics, which the regulars put a stop to right away.

As I was chatting, the boy exited the store. I told him thanks for having lunch with me and that I'll talk to him soon. He waved goodbye. One of the regulars, a woman named Maria, pointed out, "You know, it's pretty weird to have a stranger from another country come here and have lunch with one of our kids. We love that kid like he is our own, and we don't take kindly to weird strangers." Immediately on the defensive, I said I was harmless and merely wanted to talk to the kid because I love kids. I told them about how in Tanzania every kid is everyone's kid, so there's nothing foul about a Canadian having lunch with a *watoto*. To this, Maria replied, "This isn't Tanzania. This is America." I tried once more to plead my case and say I was merely misunderstood, and that all I wanted was what was best for the boy, but I could tell I had outstayed my welcome. I went back into the convenience store to buy a few more things before the drive back to Canada.

Help

I remember feeling crushed that I had given off even a scent of paedophilia in my exchanges with the boy. It didn't make sense to me. I treated him just like I would treat any kid in Tanzania or in my school placements. That didn't matter though, because "perception is everything", I reminded myself. At this point, I was exhausted emotionally and physically. I had barely eaten, hadn't drunk much water, and was mentally tired from all the ideas I had had that day. I contemplated driving somewhere and sleeping in my truck for the evening. However, as I was standing in line to check out, someone recognized me. "Jason, is that you?" It was my sister's childhood friend DJ, and she had a concerned look on her face.

She asked me what I was doing down here, and I said, "You know, scheming, changing the world, the usual." She brought her father Garry over to where I was, and he looked even more concerned. I had played baseball with his son, so I knew him since I was a child. He cared about me, and on that day, he and his daughter DJ rescued me. They said I looked exhausted and asked if I wanted a ride home. They said DJ could drive my truck, and Garry could follow us. Dazed and confused, I said sure. I paid the uncle for my items and said I would visit soon, and that I was sorry for any misunderstandings. I forgot the bag of shopping on the floor, but had the cigarettes I purchased in my pocket. DJ and I hopped in my truck and drove away.

I was drained. It didn't take us long to get to the border. I didn't realize I would have to pay duties and fees for my stereo, and they were high, bringing the US $2,000 stereo to about CAN $3,000. It took us a while to get through duties, but Garry and DJ were very patient. They could tell I was in distress and were very calming. I was too tired to rant and rave, so was mostly quiet. When we left the border and were headed home, I started to get very emotional with DJ, and even began to cry. I told her about the day, and how I had come up with these big plans to transform the town and transform my life. But I was still crushed at how the locals thought of me as a threat to their kids. I told DJ how it was obviously not my intention. I love kids, but never in that kind of a way; I love sparking curiosity, not attraction. DJ was quite comforting, and she did an excellent job of just listening. She let me talk myself out, and I was getting more tired by the minute.

When we finally reached my westside home, I thanked them very much for coming to my rescue, and told them I had just planned to sleep on the side of the road in my truck. With concern in their eyes, they said it was no problem, and didn't leave until they saw me enter my house safely. They live by my parents, and even though it was fairly late in the evening, they went straight to my parents' place to tell them what had happened. My mother would say later that Garry was very concerned for my well being, as he said I "looked lost" in the border town. This greatly concerned my parents, and they were on high alert of my behaviours afterward.

As for me, when I got home, I put the new stereo down in the living room, smoked some pot and nestled into bed. There was a message waiting for me on Facebook. It was from the boy's uncle who had found me on Facebook, most likely with the card I left with the boy. He simply said, "Stay in Canada and away from my nephew." I felt awful about the perception I had left with the locals, and I decided to reply to the message and share with him my thoughts on the day. I started by saying, "I will never return to your small town unless I am welcomed [sic]." I said, "Let me explain my bizarre behaviour ... I was dazed and confused and felt like I was in a movie. I was drawn to the simplicity of your town." Speaking to my mental health, I self-diagnosed and said, "I was clinically in a state of insomnia." I admitted my mistake, saying, "I realize now that it is not okay to be a stranger and have lunch with a random *watoto* (child) even though it was okay in Africa. I'm mad my strategy was wrong because I wanted to take that kid to the next level (whatever his definition of that is)." I ended the long message by saying, "I sincerely apologize for upsetting the community I invaded. I am not crazy, and I am certainly not a pedophile [sic]. My only intentions were to empower that boy, so he knows that the world is bigger than his small town. That's why I talked to him because I love kids and love empowering kids. I understand it's safer to banish me than become friends with me, but I hope you'll consider having me return." I left a few links to the organization I travelled with for the uncle to pass along to the boy and pressed send. The uncle would never reply.

It was 2:30am after I hit send and, feeling like I had saved the day with my message, I smoked a little more pot and drifted off to sleep. It had been an exhausting day but, overall, I thought it was a productive one. The madness was still only in the beginning.

15

22 AUGUST

Following my trip to the States, my parents were quite concerned for my well being. My mother sent my father and grandfather to check in on me unannounced. They showed up before lunch, and I hadn't been up for very long. I was working on the house, moving stuff around, trying to organize my things that were scattered in "stations" around the house. Instead of unpacking things when I first moved in, I just put everything in areas around the house to unpack later. My dad and grandfather were taken aback at how messy the house was – and it was a mess. I remember my dad criticizing me for this, and explaining it would only take ten minutes to at least take the garbage out of the house. I was a little annoyed, as he had come unannounced and was now criticizing how I was living. He was obviously worried, and got serious with me when we were in the basement of the house. He and my grandfather asked me questions about my activities, and I wouldn't give them a straight answer. I was kind of rude to my grandfather, and my dad was furious at this. Commenting on all my "change the world" plans, he said plainly, "Nobody gives a fuck about those people in Tanzania. Start being yourself again."

"What if this is my real self?" I replied, and started to cry.

My dad told me to stop crying and said, "Your behaviour is just erratic. Your mother is going to call the ambulance. We all think you're on crack or something."

This comment angered me, "I've only done acid once, and it opened my mind as it's intended to. Successful people I idolize do acid because it's helpful for your mental health."

My dad didn't really register this. Seeing that the conversation was going nowhere, he ended it with, "If you want to make a difference in this world, then start in your own backyard. Make your bed, clean your house and volunteer here in town, if you're so eager."

"Challenge accepted," I told him, and with that I finally got them to leave my house.

Ideas

With my dad and grandfather finally leaving me alone, I was free to ponder some of the great ideas I had had over the last week or so. I journaled in my phone about starting a real-estate business in the small border town I had visited. I envisioned my own shipping company out there, with my own little house near it with a shack in which I imagined myself sharing Canadian medicinal marijuana with local Americans.

I journaled about organizing my own trip to Tanzania exclusively with teachers. I would use my personal contacts there, and we would have a journey full of discovery and magic, without all the stupid rules I had been subject to. I had a detailed plan for this, with a list of all of my friends from Tanzania who would be our guides.

I talked about how our university could put on Pink Floyd's *The Wall* production for the fall. As *The Wall* is one of the most expensive concerts ever – to think our university could produce it shows how delusional I was. I even tweeted the university and the drama department about this idea saying, "We need to make this happen." No one responded, of course.

As for writing projects, I jotted down my ideas for writing columns for the university magazine, and books on "Teaching Tips and Techniques", "Facilitation Management Strategies", "The REAL Millennial Mindset", a parable of some sort and even a live-action play.

I wrote of how I would launch my motivational speaking career and money mastery programs. My thought was that I could start small by setting up a weekly show on the campus radio station, where I could rant about whatever was on my mind. I had so many good ideas about starting my personal development career that I truly believed I was starting my path towards becoming the Canadian Tony Robbins.

As I felt like an "Expert in Everything", none of these ideas felt outlandish in any sense. I even thought that I could help people fundraise a trip to the moon – it seemed an attainable goal.

With all these ideas swirling in my head, I headed to Facebook to warn people of the brilliance ahead. I made a post saying, "Save the date September 1, 2017, 12:50pm", which was the day I planned to be launch all my ideas. Some people asked what the significance was, but I was very secretive. In reality, it's ironic that I chose this date, as it ended up being my first full day in the acute psychiatry ward.

Daily Reflection

In the evening, after a day spent brainstorming and my dad showing up unannounced, I started yet another audio journal. I began with, "A happy open mind is often very kind. See! I've got original thoughts and quotes!" After discovering my own brilliance – yet again – I started a thought on copyrighting, "There should be no copyright. We should all have access to everything." I spoke about everyone's perception of me, "Literally everyone thinks I am insane. I was delirious yesterday… I wanna be anywhere but home with my parents. I am not insane."

Speaking about my mom's threat of calling an ambulance, "If they make me talk to a psychologist, I'll shrink him! I'll just flip everything on him. Everyone's got it wrong. I'd love to go to the loony bin and show everybody wrong. It's not cool that Dad thinks I'm insane and my grandparents think I'm on crack. That's insane that they think I'm insane." I got serious about my mental well being, "Maybe I am crazy, and I show a psychologist these thoughts and ask if there is any value here." I brushed that off, and said to the imaginary psychologist, "How about you come to work for me? And I'll show you how to really do your job, Mr Psychologist!" I ended with, "I'm talking to myself, and that's okay because that's how the brain works."

It was an interesting recording, because it speaks about my thoughts on my mental health and the perceptions of others. I didn't care much about what other people thought of me, and I even embraced the idea of being "crazy", because I thought that "crazy" people ran the world. Some friends came over that night and, without telling them, I recorded our conversation deep into the night, and this recording is yet another example of my rapid speech and random thought processes.

Friends

My friends Jafari and Cordelia came over to hang out. As usual, I was rambling and not letting anyone else get a word in. Jafari can be heard trying to cut me off to get a word in. When he finally did, he asked an excellent question: "Jason, who is your audience with the Master Minding stuff? What's the driving force? Who are you targeting?"

I dodged the question and continued rambling. "I'm trying to master communication," I claimed — which was ironic given I was an awful listener during this period. Jumping topics, I told Jafari and Cordelia, "My dad thinks I'm mentally ill." I told them how I was "scared" to lose this new-found energy and zest for life, which was, in fact, the fear of losing the manic energy. Speaking about my critics, I told my friends, "I don't give a shit if people think I'm crazy." Jafari and Cordelia were just listening at this point, and not trying to interject as I was getting emotional. I said the reason everyone thinks I'm crazy is because "I learned how to think like I'm on drugs when I'm sober." I thought this was true because my brain felt like it did the day I took LSD. I didn't really care about the term "crazy" as I said, "Anyone who's become successful has been called crazy at some point. Why would you wanna be average anyway?"

Earlier that day, my dad had challenged me to take a week off marijuana. I had scoffed at the idea because I had gone 16 days in Africa without it. In truth, and unbeknown to me, the marijuana was making my condition worse.

I finally stopped rambling to smoke some pot, and Cordelia told a story. However, I, of all people, told Cordelia she was talking too fast and cut her off, which resulted in us going on an 18-minute digression from her story. After I cut her off, she was trying to cut me off, to which I firmly replied, "Let me finish." I would not let anyone else speak. I was talking about how drugs have the "potential to unlock the brain" and give one "awareness". This is a ludicrous idea in hindsight, as drugs, for me anyway, were not a tool that unlocked the brain – they were a destructive force that nearly broke my brain.

Cordelia finally managed to get a word in. She was trying to tell me about the value of slowing down, and not worrying about achieving things all the time. She commented on how it was hard to have a conversation when she was the only sober one among the three of us. I replied, "I'm not fucked up. I just know how the brain works and know how to unlock memories at any moment. I have a photographic memory. I'm overwhelmed my brain thinks like this. It's overwhelming knowing that I can change the world in 52,000 hours."

I digressed to talk about my father. I was very critical of him, "I feel like Biff from the play *Death of a Salesman*." I got very emotional, and began to cry. I felt like Biff because Biff was always told by his father what he should be, and I felt that applied to me. It felt like my dad and I were very different and that he just didn't understand me. I had been hurt by our exchange earlier that day. He had even said, "You're half of me, son. Start acting like me again." I felt like doing anything but acting like my father. But it wasn't fair of me to be so critical of him, because all he was doing was trying to help in his own way. Nevertheless, I was hurt by his efforts to "straighten me out".

I told my friends, "Everyone important in my life will tell me to quit school and roll with the business ideas because they're solid." I didn't feel the need to ask anyone for this validation because in my mind I imagined them saying, "Go for it."

I got energized, displaying the ups and downs of the bipolar condition yet again, and said, "I'm sleep deprived, and I am crazy! Watch my brain go to work." I was speaking about how "it's all about communication" when Cordelia tried to speak again. I replied, coolly, "You're speaking when I'm speaking." From the recording, you can tell that Cordelia was losing her patience at this point.

I was telling my friends, "I gotta be more than a high school teacher. I have more to give," when they said they had to leave soon – it was past midnight. I ignored them and carried on rambling, "I like to pretend I'm in a play or a movie... I can speak Swahili now... Jason's not insane. Tell the world this is just how the brain works."

"Don't think that you have figured the way," Jafari replied.

"The more I learn, the less I know," I said poetically.

As I walked them to their car, I told them how I was going to "make my own bar" and that "I think I'm on to something here." As they got in their vehicle, I said to myself, "It's so hard to end a conversation." Specifically, it is so hard to end a conversation with a manic person. There had been 90 minutes of basically just me talking. It had felt like a good conversation at the time, but in reality it was just me rambling, jumping topics and being rude to my closest friends.

Another of my friends, Ross, texted me after Jafari and Cordelia had left. Talking about my social media posts, he said, "I'm trying to put the pieces of your puzzle together." I tried to explain that there was no answer to the puzzle, and that was the point. I told him, "Call me before you call the hospital. I'm not sick." Before he could reply, I texted, "My dad is so pissed." Ross replied, "Why?"

"Because I moved out real fast and have been acting very strange recently because of what I think is a mixture of insomnia and culture shock, which my parents don't understand at all. I'm fine. I literally made a million dollars. Like seriously."

Intrigued, Ross asked, "Really?"

I told him that it was my ideas that were worth millions.

Ross then bluntly said, "Jason, you gotta be on drugs right now."

Being that I had just smoked pot, I replied, "Oh, you betcha. Very creative stuff. Canada's BEST!"

To this, Ross said, "I wanna be what you're on."

I then jumped topics and randomly said, "I'm dropping out of school. Gonna start my empire."

Ross replied, "Jason, I have been in your state of mind before, and you have got to be on drugs stronger than marijuana."

"Nope. Just figured out how to think like I'm on drugs. I'm literally gonna buy a country and just make it sick," I said. It was very late at night, and I told Ross how I was "soooo tired".

Ross said I was getting "brain swirls", which I said was "literally nuts".

I casually said, "I'm not going to the States for a while. Got kicked out."

Ross replied, "WTF."

I told him I'd tell him another time as I was finally going to try and get some sleep. I had a big day planned yet again.

16

THE PROFESSOR AND *THE ROLLING STONE*

Earlier in the week, I had emailed my business professor, to see if he would like to meet up, so I could ask him some questions about starting a professional consulting business ("Holistic Solutions"). My professor is an expert in professional consulting and, surprisingly, agreed to meet with me.

Before our 10am meeting at the university, I started another audio journal. I had some more ideas for the bar I would build one day. They included "sending every second pint of beer profits to Africa" and "a bar where you can play your own music via Bluetooth speakers". Both terrible ideas, in retrospect. I came up with a new slogan for the marijuana bar, "A place to drink and think." I then jumped topics, "I am one person away from the Prime Minister," speaking about my connection to Jordie, Prime Minister Trudeau's communications advisor. Then I got angry and yelled into my phone, "Dammit Mayor! Fix this traffic. It is so inefficient, it's brutal!" Calming a little, I said, "I need to channel my energy better and control my emotions consciously." In reality, I had no control over my energy or emotions. "You know rapport better than anyone," I said. And speaking about my upcoming meeting, "More than anything, I wanna listen," which was utterly false, because all I wanted to do was talk.

After briefly explaining some of my ideas and mentioning my adoration of Tim Ferriss, my professor warned me that I might have a success bias in my business ideas. "It's not always as simple as looking at the most successful," he said. He criticized Tim Ferriss as someone who only looks at "peak performers"; my professor was warning me that I wasn't digging deep enough in my ideas to think about the negatives of launching a business, quitting school, etc. I responded with a ten-minute speech about how Holistic Solutions was all about empowering people, and that "I am a super performer/learner." I also lied and said that I was "three phone calls away from reaching Tim Ferriss." My professor politely nodded and said, "Right", "Okay", "Yeah", "Sure", "But", "Yep". I wouldn't let him get a word in. He finally got to ask an important question, "What do you hope to accomplish?"

I cut him off before he could finish, to say how it was all about helping other people, among other things.

My professor warned again, "Everything is complicated. The world is not over when you fail." He asked again, "What is your long-term goal? What need is fuelling you? Why do you want all this?"

I gave him another long-winded answer, jumped topics, and displayed, again, my rapid speech. I recall it was a scrambled answer. In the middle of it, my professor stopped me, saying he had to go and, on leaving, told me, "Remember the success bias."

My professor didn't know I had recorded the conversation. Going back over it, it is evident that I let him speak for about eight minutes of the 30-minute meeting. He was mostly concerned with my idea of quitting school because, while there have been some successful entrepreneurs that have quit school and done great things, there are probably more who have failed. Having the success bias, I ignored this, preferring to only look at the successful people, rather than the whole picture. It's interesting that my professor stayed for the whole 30 minutes, as I was quite annoying. He made some excellent points, but I continued to think only about success.

Rolling Stone Magazine

After our meeting, I had to go downtown to organize vehicle insurance, and I spotted a new coffee shop that had opened near the insurers – Sonder Café. "Sonder" is a word I learned in Arizona; it means you look at other human beings as creatures that have just as exciting and vital existences as yourself. I loved the word, and I thought it brought an awareness to me that other peoples' lives are as meaningful as my own. I was, of course, completely absorbed in my own world at the time, but I still thought it was cool that a café was named that.

I walked in and ordered some food, as I hadn't eaten yet and it was already 12:30pm. I was supposed to have met my family doctor at noon, but had completely forgotten about the appointment. I was so absorbed in the meeting with my professor and feeling so good that going to the doctor had slipped my mind. This story would probably have ended here if I had attended that appointment. Instead, there would be another week of high mania before I was to see a doctor and be admitted.

While I was waiting for my food, I came across an article on www.rollingstone.com about Roger Waters and his new tour. I was already overly excited because I had secured tickets to see him, not one night, but both nights in the big city. While reading, I got a brilliant idea, "What if I applied for a job with *Rolling Stone* and got it? I'm a writer, aren't I? Hell, I could even do an internship for free," I thought. "And imagine living in the States and working for the best music magazine in the world!" With these thoughts swirling in my head, I scrolled to the bottom of the page of the article and clicked on "Apply now." I saw the general email address to *Rolling Stone*'s Human Resources and, bouncing with energy, I opened email on my phone and began to type.

"Hello, I am a passionate, fired up 'Angry Young Man' (Billy Joel) with a plan to change the world."

I told them about reading the article on Roger Waters and being motivated to contact them. I lied, "I've learned to teach all learners. I have minors in English, social studies, and general business". I wrote, "I wanted to teach, but the classroom isn't big enough. I am an aspiring writer, author, songwriter, musician, and World Changer. My dream is to meet Roger Waters and become his *rafiki bora* (good friend)."

I asked some general questions about how I could start working at *Rolling Stone*, and finished with, "I am a man with a millennial change-happens-in-an-instant kinda plan. I wanna be the bird that spreads the word." But I wasn't finished yet. In a PS, PPS, and PPPS, I wrote, "I seriously need some help getting these ideas on-page in a more clear and concise way." "My trip to Tanzania made me question everything in North America." "I'm just a curious Canadian looking for some real answers. Looking for the Truth." And, in an audacious PPPPS, I told them about the Master Minding Facebook group, and listed seven sources for them to check out. It's been years since I wrote that email, and I am still waiting for a response.

I was probably inspired to write the email by the movie, *Almost Famous*, in which a high school kid gets a job with *Rolling Stone*, and writes about concerts and follows a band on tour. I believe I imagined the same fate for myself. With my food getting cold, I finally put my phone down and began to eat. I was so excited about waiting to hear back from them that I told the waitress about how I had just applied for a position with the magazine. I told her all about how I was a big shot and how she had just witnessed history and would be reading about this moment in a book one day. I got her to follow my journey on social media, left her a good tip and walked out of the café.

I didn't do much for the rest of the day as I had a shift with the catering company that night – my first shift since my return from Africa.

17

WASTING FOOD

On this catering shift, we were serving guests a buffet dinner of roast beef, potatoes, vegetables, salad and dessert. There was a large amount of food wasted. After the shift, I wrote some posts on the Master Minding group to explain what had happened. "My heart sank at all the food that was on the counter ready to be thrown out. What kind of images were in my head?" I remember having images of skinny children from Africa in my mind. I posted, "I won't stand for it. Not anymore." I posted some dialogue to the group from the conversation I had with the chef at the catering company.

Me: "So, hey, I just moved out, and I know some hungry housemates. Do we throw any of this out or do we repurpose it?"

Chef: "Actually, apparently, we were giving too much to [charity], so 98% is going to be thrown out."

Me: "Sorry, woah. Say that again? Are you fucking kidding me? Like I literally just got back from Africa where people are starving."

Chef: "Hey man, talk to the boss. We're rattled here in the kitchen too."

Me: "Oh, man, I need to take a break right now."

What happened after this conversation with the chef is worth noting.

My shift supervisor could tell I was upset after the conversation in the kitchen, and she let me take an extended break. I was very fired up, and I called my boss right away. It turned out to be an almost hour-long conversation that was all over the place. I expressed my grave concerns about the food waste, but I also told my boss about the struggles I was having with readjusting to North American life. I remember her being very comforting and understanding. I also remember saying that I would help co-write a book with her about her management techniques, because I thought she was such a superior manager to the ones I had in the past. While we were talking, I was pacing back and forth outside on a busy street and must have looked bizarre, my arms flailing about passionately while speaking into the phone.

We ended the conversation agreeing it would be best if I went home that night and took a break from work for a while. I could come back in a few weeks when I had cooled down and was feeling better. I was ready to quit that night, but this seemed like the better option. It wouldn't matter though, as it did end up being my last shift – when I got out of the hospital, they had filled my position. When I tried to get my job back, they didn't really want me back because of the "argument" I had with the chef. I don't blame them – they are running a for-profit business, and I had rattled the kitchen that night.

Interestingly enough, I overreacted about the food waste. The catering company actually repurposes and donates more food than any other catering business in the area. Some food has no other option than to be wasted. The owner did reach out to me over the matter, but then I ended up in hospital.

New Computer

After I had been sent home from work, I decided to swing by my parents' place because I had a package waiting for me to pick up. It was the new $1,200 computer that Quinn had said was the best in the world. I had used the wrong shipping address when I bought the computer, which is why it was delivered to my parents' place. I was excited to check it out, but not overly excited about seeing my parents. They were shocked that I had been sent home from the catering company, and we got into an argument about it while I was having a bite to eat with them. I got frustrated mid-bite, and decided to leave. My dad was angry about me rushing out of the house, but I didn't really care − I just wanted to get the hell out of there. I hopped into my truck with my new computer, and decided I really needed a toke of marijuana to calm me down. I called my friend Dylan who lives down the street from my parents, but he didn't pick up. I decided to go over there and knock on his garage to see if he was in anyway. He wasn't, but his dad Craig was. I asked Craig if I could please have some weed, as I had had a really tough night. Craig was uncomfortable with this. I proceeded to tell him all about my night, and then, getting emotional, I told him about how my dad and I weren't getting along. Craig was sympathetic to this because he had had struggles with his father too. He consoled me, and said it was too bad I was in such a tough spot. After venting for a while, I calmed down and started to feel better. I thanked Craig for his time, hopped into my truck and headed to my westside home.

When I pulled up, I saw that my neighbour Derrick was in his garage, so I popped over. I told him all about the fancy new computer I had bought, and then talked to him about living on the westside. Derrick was happy I had moved in, and we talked about how bad a neighbour my housemate had been. I reassured him again that things were changing, and I would settle him down. I even suggested how I would one day put on a free concert with my future, world-famous band to bring the community together. He thought that was a cool idea, and we called it a night.

18

SOCIAL MEDIA

Facebook

Beyond the Master Minding group, I was posting a lot of content on my Facebook page. To rationalize my large number of posts, I said that my goal was "impact" – I wanted to reach as many people as possible through social media and spread my world-changing ideas. Not many people "liked" my posts because they were long and scattered, so I began hitting the like button on my own posts, which must have looked pretty pathetic. I did have a little encouragement, however, from one friend: "This new form of posting makes for a more interesting news feed. I enjoy it." This bit of support went a long way, and #WackyWegner continued to post.

In one long post, I acknowledged people's concern for me: "Please know that I truly thank everyone for their concern in my health and I wanna say right now that I am #okay. So, stop worrying about me and worry about yourself. I'm on no drugs," which was a lie because I was smoking marijuana regularly, "I'm just using social media differently because I'm unique. I think a mile a minute and I like to type a mile a minute. So, if you don't like it leave. I am sick of people telling me what to do and how I do it, which is why I am doing my own thing. I'm not hurting anybody. I'm trying to help everybody."

There was undoubtedly concern from some people as not all of my posts were as coherent as the one above. One friend commented on one of my more erratic posts, "Is this English?" To which another friend commented, "As long as there's capital letters, he doesn't give a fuck what language it is." This comment was speaking about my regular seeding of Swahili or Spanish words in my posts. I would drop them in thinking people would understand the reference or what they meant, but as another friend commented, "You're babbling bud."

I was sick of people negatively commenting on my Facebook page, so I posted, "The sheep may unfriend me now or await the slaughtering." I said the "Night of Long Pens" was coming, meaning I would do a massive overhaul of my friends list and unfriend anyone who wasn't on board with my mission.

The Parable

On Facebook, I was also randomly posting snippets of dialogue from a story I was making up on the go. It had a main character (MC) and a spirit-like God figure (S). The spirit was purposefully confusing and supposedly wise, and would sometimes speak in Swahili.

MC: I love all of this thinking.

S: Then think quieter, ya wacko.

MC: I should listen then?

S: Yes.

MC: So, stop typing?

S: *Ndio* (yes).

The main character would try asking the spirit more questions, but the spirit said,

S: I must go now. You are interrupting my pondering, and I am interrupting your wandering.

MC: I don't follow...

S: I know you don't. That's why I am speaking to you. Continue to not follow. Lead instead. You know all the answers because you came up with the question.

MC: This is so confusing.

The spirit would act as a facilitator of knowledge and would shout in capital letters regularly. The spirit would sing song lyrics too. It would be a motivational speaker to the main character, and say encouragingly, "Good question." The main character would love the spirit and call it "The boss". I think I was trying to make the characters like Socrates and Dan from Dan Millman's *Way of the Peaceful Warrior*.

As you can imagine, this dialogue, randomly dropped into my feed, would be confusing to anyone that took the time to read it. While I thought I was incredibly clever to write a parable on my Facebook feed, it wasn't really a parable – it was just snippets of me talking to myself. The spirit character was the voice in my head, and I was the main character. I was posting my thoughts as a stream of consciousness, which I thought was brilliant. It's interesting, looking back on these particular posts, because the dialogue is a reflection of how my mind was working. I continuously had confusing or opposing thoughts in my head, and I shared them on Facebook, sometimes through this parable.

Realizing that I wasn't making waves on Facebook, I decided to take my social media talents to Twitter. I said in a Facebook post, "I just realized I've been trying to make Facebook something it's not, i.e., Twitter when Twitter was here the whole time!" I went on to tweet a massive amount in a short time. I even had two phones going, so when the battery on one phone died I was able to continue posting seamlessly. To say it was a lot of content would be an understatement – I was making close to 100 posts a day on social media.

Twitter

My first tweet during my mania said, "What follows from this moment in time on this account is The Real Me that's been bottled up. Well, somebody in Africa popped that bottle." I started my escapades on Twitter by tweeting my university and describing, in detail, my idea for putting on a production of Pink Floyd's *The Wall* in the fall. I said,

"I 100% call dibs on the lead role though of course." I tagged the university, two professors, the Student Union, the university Alumni board and *Rolling Stone*. None of them responded.

The next tweet I sent said I was "Open for business! Need a motivational speaker? Want one for a fair price?" After launching my motivational speaking career, I tweeted the President of the United States saying, "Hey @realDonaldTrump #LetsTalk. I've got an interview with @JustinTrudeau #soon #AND I'd love to hear from you and #GiveYaTheMic #WW #CC (crazy Canadian)." This tweet certainly displays some of my delusional thinking at the time as I by no means had an interview with the Prime Minister lined up in the near future, and I most certainly had no chance of interviewing President Trump. In one tweet, I asked, "Does it look like I'm lost? Or does it look like I'm finally found?"

Most of my tweets were like my Facebook posts, scattered and, at times, incomprehensible. I also tweeted a lot of short tweets all at once. This constant tweeting must have been annoying to the few followers I had, as their feed would be filled with my ramblings. But, as I tweeted the one day, "I talk fast. I write fast. I tweet fast because I think fast." I also used my Twitter account to spread the word about my health. I snarled in one tweet, "STOP ASSUMING I'M ON DRUGS". A more serious tweet read, "I don't really appreciate the word crazy. How about you say Bold instead?"

While my Twitter account was scattered and erratic, my secret Twitter account that had no followers was even more manic and erratic. I called the account @RW94147336, which is Roger Waters' initials, but had the dual meaning (at least to me) of "Rebel Wegner". My first tweet said, "This is an online book I am writing publicly. It neither starts nor finishes. It may be complete randomness, or it may be a secret account from a Brilliant Mind."

Much of the content was dialogue between the spirit and the main character, but some tweets were just thoughts. In one, interestingly enough, I come right out and say, "I'M FUCKING CRAZZZZZZZY." No one ever saw these tweets, so it was more like a personal journal. But it is interesting that I call myself crazy, because in my main account

I had said I didn't like people using that word to describe me.

With all of these erratic and scattered social media posts, my family was starting to get concerned. My sister texted me, "Ease up on the tweeting to your professors and anyone at the university. What you say on the internet is forever." My mother was most concerned, however, which is why I wrote her a massive email to explain that I was alright.

Email to Mom

In the email to my mother, I told her that I was adding her to the Master Minding group, as it would "explain my 'weird' behaviour." In addition to this, I wanted to show her my new-found creative powers, so I wrote her a poem. It wasn't much of a poem, however, rather just a list of 129 words that completed the statement "Jason is a ____". The entries included weirdo, crazy kid, artist, carpenter, English nerd, business generator, helicopter driver, philosophical storyteller, movie star, pothead, politician, consultant, rock opera creator, scientist, actor, teacher, WORLD-CHANGER, inventor, to name a few.

I told my mom that "I love a lot of things you and dad disdain... maybe I'd really just like some time to think and record some thoughts and get 'em out to the world I see in pain." I reassured her, "I'm fine. I've never felt better. I'm happy, and I'm okay." I spoke about my individuality: "I'm weird as hell. I'm abnormal. Hell, I may even be on the autism spectrum (that'd explain a lot). You keep underestimating me, but I AM POWERFUL BEYOND MEASURE! I hate the idea of being considered average. Lazy isn't in my vocabulary."

I then started writing in the third person, which was something I was regularly doing now (and which my dad hated). "Rest easy knowing that the New Jason that freaked ya out this week is gonna be a better Jason for himself, family, friends, community, city, country, world and universe (because hey Mars is 40 years away (I have the evidence lol)). I'm rambling, but this is the real Jason Wegner."

I continued to ramble, and wrote something that undoubtedly would have concerned my mother, "Maybe I'm sleep deprived, crazy, on crack and need to see a qualified professional. Or maybe I'm a smart-ass that isn't afraid to be a little rebellious and curious sometimes." Even joking about being on crack was cause for concern, because my grandparents already thought my actions were those of someone who was on crack. I continued, "I'm done not being myself. This is me. I wanna break from school so I can work and write. I wanna live. I wanna travel. I wanna do what I want." This was my first hint to my mom that I didn't want to go to school anymore. I likened my trip to Tanzania as a "jam-packed trip that was like taking a whole semester abroad in 16 days". Also, I had businesses to launch, apps to create, books to write, a podcast to run and people to see, so I didn't think I had time for school. I told my mom outright, "I need a fall semester off. It'd be best for my health." Ironically, I spent the fall semester in hospital.

I ended the email talking about how "I'm not at home anymore... free to make my own decisions and take care of myself... a big boy now". I aired my grievances with my parents, writing, "Dad has been silently (unconsciously) pushing me down to a small speck lately. And you Mom have been unconsciously 'put[ing] all your fears into me... I refuse to be the before-Tanzania-trip Jason. I'm ready to try something else. Like being a writer (hello *Rolling Stone* internship!), I like the new and improved Jason. He's more crazy, more authentic, more bold, more independent, more himself. I'm mad I couldn't share the real me to the world sooner. So, Jambo Canada! This is the new me! Don't like it? GFY! Hope this clears the air." And, with that, I pressed send.

19

25 AUGUST

Trespassing

On the morning of 25 August, I began the day with my new routine of taking a morning walk. In Tanzania, each day started with an early morning walk, and I missed it. For this walk, I ended up at the end of the road in my neighbourhood, which looked on to an open field. I decided that, like Tanzania, any area was fair game for a walk. So, around 10am, I was walking in an open field, bouncing with energy. I started a Snapchat video so I could show all of my viewers that they too could be on my level of energy. "I'm on the loose! I'm crazy!" I said, then spoke about how people kept telling me to "turn it down a notch." To that, I replied, "Fuck the notch! I turn the dial where I want. Why not be at a level ten all the time! If you need me to turn it down a notch, YOU can leave the room." I was shouting, "It's okay to be weird. Hashtag WW means Weird Wegner." Switching thoughts, I said, "I'm just the guy that wants to make some change. Just do it. Just ask." Speaking about my intentions, I said, "I'm not a pedophile [sic], or some guy looking for a buck." I ended the 15-minute rant, by imploring my followers to unfollow me, and said that I was "doing a genocide on my friends' list on social media" – meaning that I would reject anyone who showed the slightest bit of negativity. The last thing I said was, "Be yourself, and let me be me."

While I was taping this rant, my phone was buzzing with texts from my softball team's group chat. The guys were wondering what the hell I was doing in a random field, and stressed their concern and agitation about my recent posts and activities. I got into an argument right away with them and was texting a mile a minute. The team was getting annoyed and let me know it. Fired up, I said, "To hell with you guys," and quit the team. I exited the group chat and cut off my communication with them. It was a surprising move, as playing softball with my friends was one of my favourite things in the world to do, yet I tossed it aside in an instant. But I felt I had no time or room in my life for any form of negativity.

My friends from the softball team weren't the only ones texting me. My sister messaged me, "You're trespassing on private property. I wouldn't let you speak to my kids. You're not acting like a very good example."

I laughed this off, writing, "That's literally hilarious. This will be in my book one day, 100%!" She didn't reply.

I went home and began scrolling on social media. I came across a picture from a girl I used to work with and had always had a crush on. Feeling particularly bold after my morning walk, I decided to go for it and message her. I took a picture of a painting by her that I had won at the staff Christmas party, and told her that she was beautiful. I wish that had been the end of it, but I went on to send 22 more messages of nonsensical ramblings. She responded to the first message about her painting, but the subsequent 20 messages never got a reply.

A few hours later, I was on Instagram, and enthusiastically replied to every story post that was made. I "liked" every post and was craving interaction with anyone. Continuing my boldness for the day, I slid into the direct messages of who I thought were the two hottest girls at our university. One was a neuroscience student, and the other played for the women's hockey team. I made a lame attempt at flirting and sent more bizarre ramblings, sprinkled with phrases in Swahili. They both replied to some of the first messages politely, but were clearly not interested.

That night, I made a brief Snapchat video about my lack of sleep. "I've been up for like 20 hours and can't sleep." I smoked a lot of pot to try to get me to sleep, but it didn't help. I still had a lot of energy, even though I was stoned, so I posted more on Facebook. One friend tried to talk some sense into me as I continued to ramble on my Facebook wall. He said, "Insanity is when you try the same things over and over again expecting different results." He was talking about my constant Facebook posts, and my efforts to change the world through social media. I had been posting a lot of content, waiting for a response, but getting none. My friend summed me up quite well: "It seems like you took a whole bottle of caffeine pills or something." This is a terrific description of what a manic person is like. I had so much energy that I couldn't sleep, and so I took that energy to the internet and exposed my "insanity".

I virtually pulled an all-nighter and spent my time trolling different groups on Facebook run by strangers. I was very annoying, and one stranger even private messaged me telling me to F-off. I continued this behaviour until I finally drifted off to sleep, after what had seemed, to me, a productive day.

House Behaviour

During my manic episode, it undoubtedly must have been a challenge to live with me. My housemate was quite patient, however. He didn't mind the enthusiasm, and we were friends. He was starting to get annoyed, however, at all the sticky notes I had scattered throughout the house. They had quotes, ideas and random thoughts on them. Also, all my stuff was spread out all over the house. But what annoyed him most was when I took down the bathroom mirror and replaced it with a sticky note saying, "You don't need a mirror to say you look good." While this may be true, me taking the mirror down was uncalled for. But why did I do it?

While unpacking, I found an old pair of mirrored aviator glasses. I thought they looked cool. I like the idea that every time someone looked at me, they'd see themselves. I began wearing these glasses all the time. With these glasses on, I thought I could be anyone I wanted to be – I felt like an actor. I started a Snapchat video for a girl I went to high school with. Her name was Cayley, and while I always thought I was kind to her, some people weren't. She was a drama kid and, at our school, drama kids hung out only with other drama kids, and sometimes other kids would make fun of them. I wore the sunglasses and said that I was a drama kid now too, and that I was sorry that other people made fun of her. But I ended up sending it to the wrong account, so she never saw it.

I then started a video that would be available to everyone. With the glasses on, I enthusiastically told the world, "I've been a sneaky actor the whole time." I continued to rant about this idea of being an actor and explained the glasses: "I wear glasses with mirrors, so you look at yourself. Not me." When I finished the video, I took the glasses off and went to the washroom. When I was washing up, I looked in the mirror and was frightened. I looked dishevelled, as I hadn't showered in a few days, but what scared me most was my eyes. I thought my eyes looked spookily dilated, and it freaked me out. It reminded me of the horrifying and haunting image of my dilated eyes when I was on LSD. I sprinted to my bedroom to grab the mirrored glasses. I started to pretend to be one of my favourite actors, Jack Nicholson. I truly believed I was an excellent actor, but I was afraid of the mirror. With the glasses on, I carefully took down the bathroom mirror and hid it in the basement where it wouldn't hurt anybody. I put up the sticky note to remind myself that I didn't need mirrors, because there were none in Tanzania. When my housemate came home, he was wondering where the hell his mirror was, and we got into a bit of an argument about why I took it down. We came to the agreement that the mirror would stay up, but I would just wear the glasses in the house to avoid my reflection – it seemed logical to me.

Social Media Niche

Following the mirror business, my friend Mike stopped by while I was attempting to clean the garage, which was an absolute mess. It was full of garbage and stuff my housemate didn't want, and it was going to take time to clean it all up. Because I had visions of a sweet garage setup, I had taken it upon myself to clean at least one side of the garage. Mike asked me what I was doing with all my posts and videos online. I told him about my mission of changing the world, to which he replied, "I just think it's all very niche, Jason. I don't think you're reaching a very big audience." Mike was right. Everything I was doing was extremely niche. While I was expecting to reach hundreds, maybe thousands of people, I was really only reaching a handful. The support I got in my posts was minimal, but *any* bit of encouragement fuelled my fire, and so I continued.

When Mike left, I took a break from cleaning the garage and replied to some texts. My friend Stacy had texted me to point out that I was being "crazy on Snapchat". I responded, "Everyone thinks I'm on drugs, but I just understand the brain better than people understand." She asked if I was sober right then, but I didn't respond to that question. I spam texted her about 20 texts in a row, and she finally said, "Tone it down this isn't productive. I'm interested in having a conversation with you, but I need it to make sense otherwise it's pointless on my end." Most conversations with me by this time were pointless and probably frustrating for the other person. She also said, "Stop trying to ALWAYS mentor," which was another annoying trait of mine. I was continually trying to coach people and tell them how to do things, but I wouldn't listen to their suggestions. I deemed any criticism as negativity, and blocked it or them out. Stacy ended the conversation, "I think you're gonna get your ass handed to you," and she wasn't far off – that night I did almost get into some trouble.

20

TOWN FEST

After texting with Stacy, I started scrolling through Facebook; my old co-worker from the sports bar had posted that he needed a few security guards to work that night at Town Fest, which is a small-town festival just outside our city. Feeling like a Yes Man, open for any opportunity, I jumped at the chance. Recently fired from two jobs, I figured a night's work would be good for the old bank account. He said I could work the six-hour shift that started at 8pm, and I would be paid $20 an hour. I was thrilled. I showered and dug out my old shirt that said "security" from my days as a bouncer. I made it to my shift just on time.

I was to stand guard at the women's washroom area to make sure no alcohol was taken inside and that no funny business was occurring. I, of course, had my mirrored glasses on at the start of the shift, and I decided to try a "social experiment" where I would continue to wear them after the sun went down. I was also wearing a black jacket over my security shirt because I was cold. This ended up causing a scene – people were wondering what the "wacko" with aviators on was doing standing next to the women's washroom. I was being overly friendly and chatting with anybody who would listen. People were taken aback that I was wearing my sunglasses at night, but I told them I had "light sensitivity" from having too many concussions. This was an outright lie, but my boss for the night said it was okay. Eventually, the police came over because they had received some complaints about the "weirdo with the glasses", and I was not identifiably a security guard. I explained, in a friendly manner, to the officers about my light sensitivity and that I was, in fact, working. I took off my jacket, and all was good. They said I had to keep my jacket off for the rest of the shift, but thought I was doing a good job otherwise.

I treated the area I was covering like it was a sacred space. I wanted the folks that were attending Town Fest to have a great night, and I was disgusted at how many people were littering, so I began picking up garbage and cleaning up the space I was stationed at. My boss came over and said I didn't have to do that, but I insisted and said, "I'm here to add value. I can do more than stand and guard a washroom." He walked away without a problem, but my old co-worker came over and outright told me to stop because I was making the other security guards look bad.

I was having a blast that night, and I loved the attention I was getting because of the mirrored glasses. Some people found me interesting, but others were repelled. I made a friend named Kennedy, and by the end of the shift, I had two good-looking girls' phone numbers. I even helped a girl who was struggling with her sexuality to come out that night and ask another girl out. I felt like a tremendous success, and my confidence was sky-high; I felt like I could do anything.

When the shift was over at 2am, I was still full of energy. I had parked relatively far away from the venue because it had been so busy, so while I walked back to my truck, I vaped some marijuana. To say I felt great would be an understatement. I had pulled $120 in one night, got phone numbers, made friends and felt like I had helped somebody. Feeling confident in my abilities, I continued to smoke pot while I made the 45-minute drive back to my house. It was a risky and illegal act to drive while high, but I didn't care. I felt like I was driving a spaceship, and my destination was the moon. Thankfully, I didn't get pulled over or, worse, get in an accident.

Classes to Take

I still wasn't tired when I got home from Town Fest, even though it was past 3am. I decided to surf my university's website to see if any new classes available in the fall piqued my interest. I wrote the course registration number of any classes I wanted to take on a yellow notepad – by the end of the session, I had listed 129 classes. I also wrote on that notepad, "Maybe I don't need a semester off. Maybe I need a semester ON." I then got the idea of maybe not needing to go to my city's university at all – perhaps I was suited for greater things. I got the idea of going to Stanford and immediately began researching the school.

I couldn't find out how to apply, so I went on Yconic, the Canadian social media platform for all things to do with university. I posted a question about how to get into Stanford, and got a few replies. I then posted my GPA, which was 3.50 at the time, and was laughed at by one Yconic user. The platform is anonymous, so anyone can hide behind a computer screen. This member was quite rude about my aspirations for the Ivy League, and I engaged in an argument with him. He was no match for my speed typing, and I completely trolled him with a massive amount of messages. I would win the battle as he gave up trying to reason with me, and I felt good about the victory. I commented on a few more posts, encouraging people and standing up to who I thought were bullies. I then went on Facebook with the idea of the hashtag "Askari".

Askari in Swahili loosely means security. When we were in Tanzania, we were told to yell "Askari" if there was ever any danger. I became good friends with the Askari, as I regularly left my tent at night and hung out with them. I explained in a post on Facebook that if anyone feels threatened or feels they are being bullied online, they should use #Askari, and that would be a signal for me to come to their aid. I wanted this hashtag to work like the Bat-Signal worked for Batman, and I imagined myself as a superhero: The Bully Buster. It was very late in the evening, so no one replied to the post, but I thought it was a great idea.

Before I went to bed, I tried to find some bullies online to engage with and beat them down. My posts were generally random, rambling thoughts directed at strangers, but it was sometimes effective. I was becoming a pretty good troll with my nonsensical writings. I finally went to bed, feeling tired from staring at the computer screen for so long, and fell asleep feeling as confident as ever.

Sadie

When I woke up the next morning, I thought I would act on my new treasures, the two phone numbers I got the night before. The first girl I messaged that morning was named Sadie. Messaged may not be the right word, however. It's more like I attacked her with texts. While I was waiting for her to reply, I kept texting her, rambling about different topics. I told her I was "scheming my way to the Prime Minister's house", and "a motivational speaker". Then I said, "I'm not normal. You probably think I'm nuts like most people." This exchange amounted to just over 20 texts in a row with no response.

Finally, she responded saying, "Just woke up. Thanks for waking me."

I asked her how she was doing, and she replied, "Drank A LOT last night. So not sure if I'm drunk or hungover still." Confused at all the texts, she said, "I forgot your name? I was drunk, and I met a lot of people and don't know half their names."

I told her who I was and sent her about ten more texts, which she never replied to. I'm pretty sure she blocked my number as I was getting very annoying. I moved on to the next number.

Dani

I decided to change my strategy a bit and not spam text the next girl, Dani. I started asking her how she was doing, and she replied, "A little hungover and yourself?"

I said, "Fully energized and a tad frustrated, to be honest."

She asked why, and I said that was a "loaded question", and proceeded to ask her out on a date so I could explain. She said she was busy that day, so I asked if I could call her, but she didn't respond. I texted her a bit more, until she finally responded saying she worked that week but that "we can make time". From this, I was confident I had scored a date. As though I was setting up a business meeting, I said,

"Give me two time frames that work for you this week." But she never responded. I was out of new numbers to flirt with.

Town Fest Friend

Instead of trying to get lucky, I decided to text Kennedy, the friend I had made the night before. She was following me on social media, so I outright asked her, "Does my writing sound like I'm drugged out of my mind?"

She said, "Your Twitter is hella confusing more than anything."

I said, "Good, that's the point. You can't think clearly if you're running a mile a minute. That's why I write a mile a minute, and everyone thinks I'm on drugs." This was an interesting exchange as it shows another symptom of mania: not being able to think clearly. Mania is like having ten times as many thoughts as the average person, and being determined to articulate every one of them.

I was sending so many texts in a row that she finally said, "You are going to blow up my phone!" She then asked, "Do you ever let anyone else ever get a word in Jason?"

I kept texting her about random topics, and saying I was a great, benevolent person who wanted to help everybody. She finally said, "How do you help people when you won't listen?" This was an excellent question, which I danced around and ignored, and continued to spam text her. She said, "You're a very difficult person to read. You talk in riddles."

"Life is a riddle," I replied.

"You're a dork," she texted, and didn't respond to any other texts.

Friendly Concern

That afternoon my friend, Tom, sent me a message via Twitter, "Love the energy, but people are wondering what drugs you are on. If you're okay with fair reason and if you're healthy right now, brother, I think for you and your goals you need to lighten up on just the output. It's all to make the world a better place, but there is so much output it's hard for anyone following to keep up. I feel that you want to reach 80–90% of people, and you need effective numbers to change/impact what you want and become the student and life teacher that you want to be." This was a very reasonable and thoughtful message from Tom. There was no reasoning with me, however.

"I AM SOBER!" I replied – which was a lie as I had just smoked some marijuana. "I'm gonna keep being crazy and wild online literally to make the point that hey, Jason is literally sober."

Had people thought that I was sober, I would surely have been committed earlier, but most people thought I was on drugs. I told Tom, "I don't sleep. I'm too busy making a difference." He didn't reply to these messages – I'm sure he threw his hands up in despair.

My aunt Juliana was also concerned about me and sent me a message. I replied, explaining about why I took drugs, "I think marijuana is medicine for my pain… I can hallucinate on-demand soberly." I remember trying to lucid dream, or hallucinate on demand, at night when I couldn't sleep, but I also experienced real psychosis – a scary state, in which you lose touch with reality and can sometimes even hallucinate – a few times during my manic episode.

I concluded my message to my aunt with, "It's so awesome that people think I am crazy because I think they're too lazy." My aunt was very supportive, and just wanted to make sure I was okay and not touching any dangerous drugs. When I told her, "I wanna go to Stanford for grad school," she said that anything was possible. While I don't think her concerns for me were fully allayed after our chat, we did end the conversation on friendly terms.

While I was busy sending out all these messages, I, once again, forgot to eat dinner. And I actually forgot that I was supposed to eat dinner at my parents' place because my sister was in town. My family was disappointed I missed it, and my sister was a little upset I didn't bother to show up. I told them I had been busy and got lost in my "work".

Later in the evening, a friend came over to hang out. He wanted to try some of my medicinal - grade marijuana. We smoked some, and he was so impressed that he asked if he could buy some from me.

Not wanting to turn into a drug dealer, I told him that I would not accept money from him but would be willing to trade the marijuana for something else. He asked what we could trade, and I told him I needed a toaster. He agreed, so I gave him the marijuana and he said he owed me a toaster. I later completely forgot about the trade as I was quite inebriated at the time of the deal, but my friend did deliver me a toaster eventually – and it was a pretty nice toaster.

After my friend left, the evening turned into night, and, before I knew it, it was four in the morning. While sitting in the backyard, high, I got the brilliant idea to send my ex-girlfriend an email. We hadn't spoken since we had broken up two years prior, but I thought that moment was the perfect time to reconnect.

It was a mess of an email. It started as a "poem", but was really just me filling in the blank to the statement "I know___"; things like "I know you think I hate you", "I know I hurt you", and "I know you enjoyed our time together". After the long "poem", I rambled a bit before saying, "Here's more confusing writing to make you think I am insane. Please don't call the ambulance to take me away for being 'crazy' lol (like my mom literally thought of doing)." I explained, "I'm not crazy. I'm just tired of being lazy with my inner self and mental health." I rambled some more, jumping topics, recalling memories and repeated, "Seriously, I'm not insane." It was 5:45am and I was still typing the massively long email. It was mostly stream of consciousness writing, and I finally concluded with "… get in touch with me when YOU are ready. Or wait to see me on TV lol." I hit send at nearly 6am, and was exhausted. I felt like I had poured my heart into the email, and felt good that I had finally gotten something off my chest.

Phished from India

Amazingly, I still did not go to sleep after this email. I went to bed and began searching for videos to watch. I was still pretty stoned. I started searching banned TED Talks, and stumbled upon some conspiracy theory videos. These videos fed into my paranoia, and I remember vividly one video felt like it was talking directly to me. I was high and sleep-deprived, so my mind was quite vulnerable to irrational ideas.

One such irrational idea was that North America was full of spies and people that could not be trusted. The thought that I may need to live in another country popped in my head. I saw that my German relative Heidi was on her Facebook chat, so I thought I would get some information about visiting Germany. This resulted in me looking at flights, asking how much money I would need to stay there, and fantasizing about leaving that week. Heidi said I was welcome any time, and I nearly took her up on that. I was a flight risk from then on, and if I hadn't been hospitalized when I was, who knows where I would be right now.

After chatting with Heidi for nearly an hour, I went to a few "inappropriate" websites. After a few clicks, my computer shut down all its controls and said a virus had been detected. It was now nearly 7:45am. As my computer was brand new, I hadn't yet put any virus protection on it. The screen told me to call a 1-800 number, which I did. Being completely sleep-deprived, I ended up giving the woman on the other line, who was in India, my credit card information. I paid US$500, they took control of my computer remotely, made some changes and "fixed" my computer by putting in their antivirus software. It didn't dawn on me right away that something was wrong with this picture, but when they were finished, I was outraged. I called them back and demanded my money back. They refused. I checked my online banking, and the money had already left my account. I called my mom in distress at 8:30am, and she told me to immediately cancel my credit card and ask the bank what I should do. The bank advised I try to speak to a manager at the antivirus software company and explain my sleep-deprived state. They said, if that didn't work, they had a small claims division that may be able to help. I called India again, and it took nearly an hour of pleading my case while riding the rollercoaster of bipolar emotions – I was angry, sad and distraught all at the same time.

Finally, a manager said, because they had "performed a service", a full refund could not take place. But the new security they put on my computer could be refunded for US$350. I cut my losses and took the deal. I was exhausted. I called my mom to tell her what had happened, and she advised me to sleep. Around 10am, I finally fell asleep, wholly depleted.

21

MR PSYCHOLOGIST

Through my mom's benefits at work, she was able to schedule a session for the family with a registered psychologist, Dr Kerry Bernes. We also managed to bypass the waiting list as Dr Bernes is a friend of Trevor. My mom said the session was more for her benefit, because she was struggling to come to terms with the "new Jason", but I was by no means reluctant to attend the session. I was confident that seeing a psychologist would finally quiet the critics of my behaviour and let me live my life. I thought I was going to school the psychologist and "shrink him". Before the meeting, as I was waiting for my parents to pick me up for the appointment, my cousin Spencer texted me with concern, "Can I ask what all the very confusing statuses are about? Like what's up bro, they don't make any sense. Did you hit a blunt too hard or what!?"

I replied, "I'm woke. Am I crazy to think society is sick of being lazy? Why do you care about my ramblings anyway?" I continued to spam text and ramble to my cousin, "My dad's a hater and my mom's scared. Did you know at Town Fest the cops checked up on me, but I helped a girl realize she was gay?"

After 53 texts in a row, my cousin finally said, "Dude, stop." Another 137 texts later, he said, "Sorry phone died." His phone probably died because I had sent him 192 texts to his eight texts in 30 minutes. The poor guy was just trying to check up on me, but my speed-texting nearly blew up his phone.

We had to wait a few minutes for Dr Bernes. I had decided that I would secretly record the session, so I could use it against the psychologist if he tried to take me away to the hospital – it would be proof of my sanity. I sneakily hid my phone under the table and hit record.

In the recording, you can hear me laughing before Dr Bernes arrived. I believe I was laughing in disbelief that I was in a shrink's office. Dr Bernes welcomed us, and I introduced myself, "I'm Jason. I've seen you around the school. The school of cool!" In addition to his private practice, Dr Bernes is a professor at my university. To start, he asked for our basic family information and history. After that, he asked me a simple question to which I gave a very long answer.

He asked, "What are you doing right now, Jason?"

I said, "I am living. I just got back from Tanzania. I'm going to work for Uber and Skip the Dishes, and I started my writing career yesterday. I started writing books. Multiple projects on the go. Moved out recently, too. Loving it. I like being weird. Stream of consciousness writing is my specialty."

Dr Bernes just nodded and said, "Mhm," while I continued to ramble on.

"I went to Hogwarts this summer. That's what Tanzania was like. I've been testing people all week, and I've been purposely confusing to see if people will pass my test and ask me if I'm okay and I tell them I'm great. See, I don't need to listen to the haters, and I've got a lot of haters." I then told him about my "sunglasses experiment" at Town Fest. Jumping topics right away, I told him I had dropped all my classes and combed through all the courses the university offered and wrote down what I was interested in. Next, I said, "We're all kids, and I'm ready to scream my kid out of me. Maybe summer camp should be longer than 16 days."

To this, Dr Bernes finally said, "I'm not following." I explained to him, "Sixteen days was how long Tanzania was." This got me on the topic of Tanzania, and I rambled on about that for a while. I told him about my business partner Quinn and about all the emails to important people I sent. I told him, "I understand the brain a lot." I got emotional talking about being friends with people who don't have friends. The ups and downs of the conversation was bipolar disorder on full display.

I casually mentioned that I had been fired from The Jungle, and said, "I wanna be Tim Ferriss. Why not?" Talking about using emotions, I said, "When you get angry, you get thinkin'. And when you get thinkin', you get answers. And I think we're all after answers." Jumping thoughts again, I said, "I'm super fed up with people saying they don't want to fucking hear me. I'll write it down then... I'm done telling people things. I'm just going to show them. I'm crazy, weird, wacky because I want kids to be like that. It's okay to be different." With me putting on this display of thoughts and scrambled thinking, I believe my dad started to tear up in disbelief that this was his son talking – he was shocked.

Dr Bernes tried to keep us on at least one topic and asked, "How did you like Education 1000?"

I replied, "I loved it. I was battling, but one day wrecked it all. I let one person tell me I wasn't good enough. One Madame President, the lead role in my play that I've already got written, because I wrote a play in Africa, because I'm allowed to be a writer here and I realize that now." This answer clearly shows how my mind would race. I couldn't answer a simple question because I couldn't have a single thought. I had many thoughts racing in my head, competing with each other for attention. Breaking down this answer, I talk about school, then about my teacher mentor, then about the play and how I'm supposedly a writer. Dr Bernes was, understandably, confused, so he asked, "Who is this person you are talking about?"

"My teacher mentor that I shadowed. She was an evil woman... she was a monster," I replied.

"So, you said you repeated Education 1000, how did that go?" Dr Bernes asked.

"It changed my life. My new teacher mentor was phenomenal." I was starting to get emotional again, and I was talking extremely fast.

Dr Bernes tried to keep on the topic saying, "Did this experience tell you that you wanted to continue in education?"

"No. No, it absolutely didn't. It told me that I wanted to do so, so much more. That's why I dropped all my classes. I want a blank slate. That's why I love my new place. It's a blank page. Nobody's telling me where to put my f-ing lawnmower or where to place my shoes. They taught me *kupenda* in Africa. It means love. *KUPENDA*. Fun to say."

I continued with this long-winded answer, "I'm interested in tonality. Linguistics, psychology, neuroscience. I'm interested in how you're sitting, and he's sitting. Interested in pacing and leading. Interested in you shaking your head right now and how you're doing this thinker thing with your fingers. Interested in your chair. I'm a motivational speaker. And actor. I'm pretending to be an actor right now." I then jumped back to Tanzania, "Somebody told me I can't go back to Africa and that nobody gives a shit about them over there. Well, I said, okay you want me to show ya? I'll show you how many people care. I'll show you that the people in my head right now care because I've got those voices. I'm not schizophrenic. I'm not insane. I'm happy. I found enlightenment, sorry." I went on to end with, "I think I've spoken enough about my story and I think I've proven, I hope I've qualified, as Neil Strauss would say, that this is me. This is the me that I've been shouting out and everybody's been telling me to tone it down. Just tone it down."

It sounded like I'd wrap up there, but I continued to ramble on for a while, and Dr Bernes just let me speak until I tired myself out. Without interruptions or questions, I continued my rant. "I smoke pot because I think too much. It's doctor-prescribed, and I need it. I've got a powerful brain and a powerful memory. I can go wherever I want, anytime. I have a photographic memory... so yeah to go back to the question, I don't wanna be in Education anymore." I told him about the podcast, and then jumped back to what I wanted to be, and made the bold statement, "I wanna be a professor of everything." Dr Bernes mildly chuckled at this.

After my professor of everything comment, I started to talk about the situation with my family. "At home, I feel like I can't be myself. I'm literally acting insane, being crazy because I'm tired of being lazy. I'm crazy on purpose because I'm sick and tired of people being lazy and just assuming things instead of asking. That's my point. So, that's all I had to say. I'm glad I got that off my chest. I hope you folks understand me a little bit better. Feels good to be me. We need more people to be okay with being themselves. We need more people to be kind because you can't rewind. You can't rewind the hate. All you got is today. And I'm tired of wasting it because I've only got 50,000 hours left in this decade and I've got a shit-ton of projects to do."

Bridging to another random thought, I said, "It's amazing how the mind works, and it's so mysterious how this mind works because how am I still talking this fast? How do I have all this energy? Well, it's because energy is all around us." I casually mentioned how I was going to the moon one day, to which Dr Bernes said, "Would be cool." He had long ago put down his notepad.

Dr Bernes already had the answer to why I was talking so fast and why I had so much energy – I was in a manic episode and I had bipolar I disorder. He had figured it out pretty fast because I was displaying all the signs: rapid thoughts, rapid speech and high energy.

We were nearing the hour mark of the session when I said, "Everybody's blind. I'm trying to make them see, and I've been scared shitless walking into a shrink's office thinking he's gonna take me away in the ambulance because I'm a lunatic, because nobody's actually asked me, 'Hey Jason, what's on your mind?' By the way, thanks for wearing blue. Did you know it was my favourite colour? Of course, you didn't. But anyways, I like other people to speak because I've said enough."

I was truly finished speaking, and Dr Bernes asked my mom what her thoughts were. She said, "I'm concerned with his enthusiasm and how he's spreading his word. I understand he's got a lot of thoughts on his mind, but I don't see a flow to it. It's very erratic. He was speaking at this rate when he got home."

My dad then chimed in, asking my mom, "What's the first thing he did when he got home?"

I answered for her, "I smoked some pot, and goddammit it felt good."

My dad elaborated on his perspective of that day. "We had picked up dinner, and it was on the table, and he felt it was more important to smoke pot than to sit down for dinner for 20 minutes after we had just driven two hours to pick him up. He just right away, immediately, went to the shed to smoke pot. Then when I came out to say something, he snapped at me. It just concerned me. I didn't understand the urgency, after speaking for two straight hours, that he just ran to the shed to smoke pot then rejoin us."

Dr Bernes asked, "How was he before the trip?"

My dad replied, "He seemed relatively the same type of person. Seemed like he was working hard, maybe cheating himself a bit on sleep. He had a concussion about three weeks prior to the trip. Seemed to be doing okay though."

"So, the energy that he has today, is that different or the same before the trip?" Dr Bernes asked.

"Oh no, this is probably five, ten times more. Like every conversation, it's elevated, like what we've seen here." My dad then turned to me and asked, "My question to you, son, is that you have all these goals, that you want to be a leader of this and a leader of that, but if you look at your social media it's... who would want to follow you? And if you think that's funny, to me it's concerning, because the people following you, like, what are they thinking? There's a lot of people that could facilitate your career moving forward, and they see this stuff, and it makes no sense. People are asking me, and I don't know what to say. It's uncharacteristic. It bothered me how you treated your grandfather the other day, and I'm scared for you to talk to my dad... You were found wandering aimlessly at the border. I am concerned for your welfare... When you're talking it's very hard to get a question in. People are losing faith in you. There's no structure to your thinking. It pains me, son, that someone who was so buttoned-down and organized is acting this way. The guy before had a plan, and I thought my kid was gonna be somebody, because people follow him by example – he leads by example. Work ethic, superior grades, behaviour, ability to start jobs and move to the top very quickly, those aren't the skills many young people have... it's like you want to flush it all away."

At this point, we were well over our time, and Dr Bernes had to check his door for the next client. He said he had to run to his next session but wanted to book another session with us. I asked, "Do you have any micro-closure here or like what's next? Do me, Mom and Dad continue that week-long break from each other that I was ready to ask for?"

Dr Bernes said he agreed with that, and said we should meet in a week to "flush this out a bit more." My dad was quite emotional after giving his speech. Seeing that it didn't really move me in any way must have made him sad. I felt after that session that nothing was wrong and that, if anything, I had proven my sanity, and I had the recording to prove it.

As we were walking out, my mom asked me about my doctor's appointment that I had missed and rescheduled. I told her I planned on going, but my dad asked, "Do we have to go check to make sure you go? Can we trust you to go there? To look after yourself?" I reassured them that I was a big boy and could look after myself. They offered to drive me home, but I lied and said I was meeting a friend downtown for dinner and that I'd walk there. They agreed to let me go, and we parted ways.

I extended the recording with a voice memo to myself after my parents had driven away. I said that this recording was an invaluable resource. I then asked myself, "Wow, what day is it? I haven't seen a clock or a mirror for days. But I'm having a blast. I'm unshakeable!" I then contemplated going to Duncan's Pub, which would have been the first time I had entered the building since being fired. I thought it would show some real confidence. But I was feeling some anxiety, and my brain was saying it was a bad idea. I asked myself, "Why the fuck would I want to go there anyway?" and turned round.

I said to myself, "Maybe you are crazy. Maybe that's the point. Maybe you'll be prime minister one day. Maybe you're delusional! But why can't I be a metaphysicist? I understand it better than all of you. Hell, I'm gonna smash metaphysics." After that, I talked about one of my genuine fears: "I'm kinda scared of getting hit by a bus. I mean John Lennon got shot, and I'm speaking like John Lennon." Moving onto my aspirations, I said, "I'm trying to be a professor right now. Because I wanna be a professor. I don't wanna be an education student. I wanna be an everything student."

I end the recording, saying that I'm ready to talk to some strangers at the bar and that I should "keep wandering, keep wondering and start sondering. Keep sondering and get pondering." By this time, I was wandering the downtown area, and the night was far from over.

Street Rant

On my way to the bar, I stopped at the rainbow crosswalk in our downtown district and decided to start a Snapchat video available to all. I began pacing back and forth in the street as traffic whizzed by and spoke passionately into my phone. "Be okay with being crazy. Rather crazy than lazy!" I said to the Snapchat viewers. Then, pointing to the rainbow crosswalk, I said, "I love all people! *Kwaheri* [goodbye] to the haters!" At this point, people in the street were laughing at me, and a few cars honked their horns; I took this as encouragement, however, and continued to pace back and forth.

I kept my rant going. "I don't need drugs, I need hugs! See, I get people to question things. So, if you're sick of Wegner rants, unfollow me." I began to walk towards the bar after a ten-minute rant near the crosswalk. I was still videoing myself as I walked down the street when I recognized somebody. It was a tall, lanky, friendly looking fellow I had seen at the bar many times at karaoke. I had also seen him around school. I wanted to prove to my Snapchat viewers that the world isn't a scary place, so I attempted to befriend this man. Luckily, he was extremely kind. As he was finishing his smoke, I told him how I had recognized him and introduced myself. Full of energy, I asked if he would be in a Snapchat video I was making for kids. He agreed, and I started recording again. "You can literally make friends with anybody kids! Isn't that right Todd?"

He said, "Yes, you can make friends with anybody."

Thrilled I had made a new friend, I asked if he wanted to have a pint at the sports bar I used to work at. He said he was headed home, but there was karaoke on at another bar near his house and asked if I wanted to go. Always open to an opportunity, I emphatically said yes and hopped in his car. We began talking on our way to the bar and found out that we had a lot in common. We were both huge Pink Floyd fans, students at the university and marijuana enthusiasts. He asked if I wanted to skip the bar and go to his place to smoke some pot instead, and I said that was a great idea. First, we had to stop for gas and being that I skipped dinner, I hopped out to buy a snack when we got to the gas station. While he was pumping the gas, I thought that I would start our new friendship with a gift. When Todd was done pumping the gas, I told the gas station clerk that I would pay for it. I forgot to buy a snack, but did pick up a fidget spinner, which was all the rage at the time. Todd was shocked that I had paid for his gas and thanked me graciously. He said he'd return the favour with some of the best weed in town.

Todd fixed himself a drink, showed me his house, and we eventually went to his office where the weed was stashed. I took a massive bong toke, and the weed instantly hit me. I was taken off guard at how powerful it was. He said it was strong stuff, and it did feel stronger than my medicinal stuff. We talked for a while, but I told him I needed to walk around a bit as I wasn't feeling very good. When I got to his living room, I had a hallucination. I remember seeing the colours yellow and red in my line of vision, and then some of my favourite celebrities emerged in the picture. Tony Robbins was there, Oprah, some family members, and what I thought was Jesus Christ. It was a complete break from reality, and crazier than any hallucination I had ever had before. Todd, concerned, tried to reel me back, asking if I was okay; I said I needed to sit down. The hallucination was over, but its image is still clear in my mind to this day.

What I had just experienced was psychosis, and *everyone* who uses marijuana is at risk of experiencing it. Some people, like myself, are more vulnerable than others, but it is a real risk of the drug. I told Todd that I needed to go home, as I wasn't feeling very well at all. He apologized for the bad trip I was having and said he would drive me home. I started to come down from the high as we got closer to my house, and I thanked Todd for the night's adventure. We agreed to meet up again sometime, with me supplying the weed instead of him.

I was lucky I had met such a nice person, as that night could have truly turned bad. Getting into a stranger's vehicle and doing drugs with them is a prime example of my risky behaviour. Experiencing psychosis was certainly scary, and I'm fortunate I made it home safe.

The night was young, however, as it was only around 10:30pm when I got home. My housemate wasn't in, so I had the place to myself. I decided to start yet another Snapchat video from my living room.

When I started the video, I was crying. I said, "I'm not a drug addict. I'm a love addict." Switching emotions quickly, I began shouting into the camera, "WAKE UP! YOU CAN BE HAPPY WITHOUT DRUGS! I'M SOBER AND INSANELY FUNNY AND HUMBLE. GET OFF MY CASE! AM I ANGRY? OH, YEAH!" Changing tempo, "Am I sad? You better believe it. Why? Because no one's listening. They're mad that I am loony or crazy when seriously, seriously all it is, is a fire in my belly that says I DON'T DO LAZY!" This rant is basically a conversation with myself and should have been a voice recording. Instead, it was broadcasted to all of my friends on Snapchat, and while some did "snap" me or message me to ask what was going on, I ignored them and continued with the rollercoaster of a video for a total of 97 minutes.

I commented, "I keep getting lost in my thoughts." I began to tear up and said, "I'm not trying to be a bad person or a wacko. I just care about helping people. Money doesn't change the world, people do. It's better to be crazy than lazy." I began ranting about how art matters and then, randomly, about Scientology and Tom Cruise. I told the imaginary audience that I was a poet and "I'll help you fundraise to the moon". I was very emotional throughout, and I thought, "Maybe this rant will go viral." I repeated to myself that I was "still not insane". I told everyone, "I'm not crazy… I can give you financial advice. All kinds of advice!… I can be a preacher. I'm invincible now!"

The video is a terrific display of a stereotypical bipolar person. I go from sadness to anger to passionate optimism within seconds. My phone finally died about 45 minutes into the rant, but my backup phone was fully charged, so I continued to pace back and forth in my living room, ranting into my phone.

I told the crowd, "Stop bashing people for being themselves… I may be on the autism spectrum." Cognizant of my scattered thinking, I said, "I am rambling, but I've got energy. I've had hardly any sleep… I'm gonna meet Eminem. I'm friends with Leonardo DiCaprio in the future as well." Shouting in my house, ranting in the dark, I honestly looked and sounded insane. This video was an example of me being in a prime state of mania. I ended the video saying, "Kids don't hate. They appreciate. I don't want you to see me until you hear me. Everyone's a kid, and I've got the plan to get lost in Germany already laid out. What you call depressing, I call powerful. I am confusing for a reason." And with that, the 97-minute broadcast was finished.

It was now around midnight and, amazingly, I was still not tired. I was running on less than five hours' sleep, and it had been a busy day and night. Restless, I decided to go for a night walk. I left my phones at the house, and began walking the alleys of the neighbourhood. I saw some trash lying on the ground, so I picked it up. Then I got the idea of cleaning up the entire alley. Like I did in Tanzania, I picked up all the trash I could. I even walked into peoples ungated backyards and picked up trash. I felt like I was making the world a better place, one piece of trash at a time.

I did this for nearly an hour. When I got home, I had a text waiting for me from my dad. He had sent me two texts earlier, but I hadn't been paying attention to my phone. At 10pm, he had asked, "Did you get home okay?", and at 12:45am he had texted "#worriedaboutmyson". My sister had seen the street rant and that I had gotten in a stranger's car. She was very concerned and told my parents, which is why my dad was texting me. I decided to smoke a little pot before I replied. At around 3:45am, I texted my dad saying, "I found what grandma calls God. I read the Bible, and I'm sober." Both were outright lies. At 4:20am, I texted, "What do you want from me? Do you want me to be happy? Because I am. Do you want me to be sad? Because I am. I wanna reach 19 million students. I could be a preacher. I'm at the top of the 1% and it's magical. I have access to all the riches in the world. You just don't see it yet. I'm not crazy, but I am a philosophical writer." Five hours later, my dad replied, "Thanks for responding. I love you, Jason... talk soon."

22

THE VOW OF SILENCE

Mental Health Line

Even after our appointment with the psychologist, my mom was insisting that I call the emergency mental health line, as she still thought I was ill. So, on the morning of 29 August, I called the number. A woman answered and asked how she could help. I told her that she was a valuable resource for people in need, but I was not one of them. I told her I was calling because my mother wanted me to, and I wanted her to get off my case. I explained to the woman how I had gone to Africa and come back with some reverse culture shock, how I had been frustrated with my family and moved out. I said I was an entrepreneur and writer, and my family didn't understand me. She was very comforting, and said I just needed to give my family some time to understand things better. She said I was handling everything well, and we ended the friendly conversation at that.

The mental health line couldn't tell that I was severely mentally ill and in a manic episode, because, at times, it was hard to detect. I wasn't exhibiting symptoms all the time, and could just seem to be a highly efficient person.

However, on this day, the scales tipped, and I became a walking mental case. It started with another ranting Snapchat video.

The Rant

I was fired up after the emergency call, and ready to talk to the world. I had taken the call as another example, in addition to the psychologist's appointment, of someone in the mental health field saying there was nothing wrong with me. I put on my aviator mirrored sunglasses and began the video in my living room with Pink Floyd music blasting in the background. I spoke about how no one had been listening to me, and that it was time for me to start showing people. "Tired of the hashtag TRUTH?" I asked my viewers, "STOP LISTENING then, because you aren't hearing me anyway! So, LEAVE, and you may return when YOU are ready."

I concluded the video by announcing a 200-day Vow of Silence. I declared that I would not speak for 200 days, and would only use non-verbal communication. I told them I was doing it for the kids that don't have a voice, and that I wanted to make a statement. I imagined the future newspaper article that would be written about my campaign: "The man that could not shut up lost his voice."

I began by writing in blue pen on the white shorts I had been wearing for the last two days. I scribbled hashtags like, #SEETHECHANGE, #WEARESILENT and #doingit, and phrases, "JustAsk", "KUPENDA" and "Peace is easy". I wrote questions like "What is time?" and, "This is nice, hey? Scary but you're an Askari Warrior!" And reminders, "Sonder Wonder Ponder", "slow down", "just breathe", "words matter". Twenty minutes later and my filthy white shorts were full of blue ink, and I was out of writing space. So, I moved on to my arms and legs.

More hashtags were written on my legs, and on one spot on my upper thigh I wrote, "TRY AGAIN", and this was where I would strike a line every time I broke my Vow of Silence. After a few hours, I had nearly ten strikes on my leg. Most of the writing is complete nonsense, but in one spot, I wrote, "@RollingStone #CANYOUHEARMENOW?" My thinking at the time was that my Vow of Silence campaign would gather national exposure and my *Rolling Stone* application would magically shoot to the top, and I would have a job with the magazine when the vow was over.

After I had finished painting my shorts and body in blue ink, I checked my phone to find multiple texts from a few friends. My friend Willy asked, "What in the world are you up to Jason?"

I sent a genuinely bizarre reply, "See, I am God, Willy. You are my son. I'm crazy."

The next text came from my friend Chase Bell, who gave me some encouragement: "I'm loving it brother, keep it up! I'll reach out when I'm in a slump, and you can fire the kid up. Your shit makes no sense, but somehow it does make sense. I've read every tweet and every status, man, grabbin' life by the balls inspires me. Love ya #ww."

Another positive text came from my friend Dylan, "Love the Snapchat story, my friend. Some great messages there. Here's why I love you as a person, Jason. You're unique, you don't let people tell you how to be or act, you're pushing for change in the right direction for yourself and this world. What you're doing isn't actually hurting anyone, people are so offended by what you're doing because their brains aren't ready for these big ideas or movements, their minds physically can't think these things are possible. They don't want to stand out."

Standing out was the whole point of the Vow of Silence, and I was pumped from my friends' encouragement. I felt in my heart that I was doing the right thing and for a great cause.

Lunch with Dad

After I had launched the Vow of Silence, my dad had offered to take me out for lunch. Given that it was nearly noon, and all I had had for breakfast was a banana and some Nutella, I happily agreed. However, I warned him that I would not be speaking during the entire lunch. I briefly explained the Vow of Silence I was taking via text, but told him I would explain on paper what I was doing. To say my dad was concerned when he picked me up would be an understatement.

With writing all over me and not saying a word, I hopped in my dad's car with my journal and pen. My dad was confused, so I wrote down on my notebook, "I've been selfish. I'm taking a Vow of Silence for the kids I saw that 'no one gives a fuck about'. I'm showing those kids I care because they're my friends, okay?" My dad nodded his head, and we drove away. We stopped at the bank first to provide them with my change of address. I entered the bank with my mirrored sunglasses on and my journal. My dad asked me to "be normal"; I went to the bank teller with my journal and wrote down the services I needed. It was relatively easy, but I could tell people were staring at me – and I must have looked bizarre with writing all over myself. I emphatically explained my campaign via paper to the bank teller and even gave her my "mobile business card" and social media information. We left the bank, and I think my dad was relieved.

McDonald's wasn't very far from the bank, and my dad said I could stay in the car while he went and got us our food. I wrote down my order, and he went inside. The moment he left, I hopped out of the car and lit up my one-hitter of marijuana and smoked it in the parking lot. I didn't want my dad to see I was getting high, but I thought the greasy fast food would taste better after a smoke. He caught me, though, and wasn't too impressed.

We drove to a nearby park with picnic tables. There was one empty one and one occupied one, and I suggested we sit with the strangers and make new friends. My dad said no, which upset me, but he snuffed out my disappointment by saying he wanted a one-on-one lunch with his son.

Because I wrote down my responses during this lunch, I still have the dialogue, and it certainly shows my mania at its peak. My dad asked what happened at The Jungle, and I simply wrote, "I gave that Jungle job up." I asked if I could have a smoke, to which my dad said no. I wrote, "I wanna smoke (cigarettes) because I'm stressed." He asked me to just speak, but I wrote, "I will speak when people will listen/want to. You were right. I need help." My dad kept trying to get me to speak, so I wrote angrily, "I can't talk, you keep asking me to talk. I will leave if you keep testing me. I am not ready for these tests. Just you talk..."

please, this is so hard. I know this is weird and stupid, but a few kids like Wacky Mr Wegner, and I just wanna make them smile. I still wanna be a great teacher, but I want to be a professor. English Prof 100%. I can and will do this, so smile and enjoy our lunch because I am. Writing is working, dad, and I will show you I AM fine."

My dad tried to show patience, but he couldn't wrap his head round my Vow of Silence. I told him, "If this town is too mean and won't understand I will leave. My head knows. Our relatives support me. $700 one way to explore and write in silence in Germany. I will go there when the time is right. I feel like this town needs to see me, not hear me speak. They don't understand." I then told him that I was doing this for the organization I had travelled with, and that the Vow of Silence campaign was my ultimate goal and focus now.

My dad had told me previously that I needed to stop talking and start doing, so I repeated his words to him, "No one wants to listen to me, so I am showing them." I reassured him that I was "very happy and content" right then with him there. But in the next strike of the pen I wrote, "I do this to understand. To understand the pain." My dad was distraught by all of this and began to tear up. So, I wrote, "Cry tears of joy, silly, your kid found that God guy." At this, my dad said he needed a second and, with tears in his eyes, he got up and took a walk to the trees nearby. He was very emotional, and I can only imagine the thoughts going through his head, *What happened to my boy? Is this really my son?*

I got up too after a few moments, and walked to the top of a hill and looked down on my dad by the trees. I remember feeling like God, and that I had cast a shadow of pain on my father that he needed to experience. I went over to him and, with tears, he said, "I just wanted to have some fucking hamburgers with my son." I gave him a big, silent hug and a few pats on the back. We went back to the table, and our conversation continued.

I wrote, "Dad, please see that I'm old enough to challenge. To challenge all. I AM ½ of you. What do you SEE? I'm part of the good guy's dad, and I'm gonna change the world. You heard it first." My dad tried to say something to get me back to reality, but I was getting frustrated, "NO, YOU DON'T GET IT STILL! This is for ONLINE

Mental Health." My dad was exhausted by this point, so he decided it was time for us to go.

My dad had tear streaks on his face – it was a tough day for him; I was terrifying him with the Vow of Silence nonsense. He had simply wanted a normal lunch with his son after the previous night's tense meeting with the psychologist. I look back on this day in shame. I couldn't help myself for behaving this way because I was in mania, yet thinking about how I made my dad feel saddens me.

The Counsellor

After my dad dropped me off I looked at my phone and saw I had a missed call from a number I didn't recognize. They had left a text message: "I am connecting because my boss received a referral this morning."

"How can I be of aid?" I replied, thinking this was a client for my consulting business.

"It's actually about you seeing him for counselling."

I was excited that someone would want me to counsel them, but frustrated that I couldn't speak because of the Vow of Silence. I briefly explained that I couldn't talk, but could certainly listen and give written advice.

The person clarified that her boss was a counsellor and was wondering if I wanted to talk to him. I replied, "Oh I'm sorry I thought you wanted me to counsel him. I'm a mentor." The person asked for confirmation that I did not want to see the counsellor, and I said I didn't, because I was perfectly fine.

My Housemate's Little Party

That night my housemate invited some girls over to hang out. They knew who I was, but hadn't seen me in my manic episode. I remember them looking shocked when they saw me with writing all over myself and wearing mirrored sunglasses in the house. Because I couldn't talk, I mostly hung out in the garage smoking pot while they were in the kitchen. I was tired, but couldn't fall asleep, so I attempted to lucid dream, which is consciously trying to dream while you are awake. I wanted to be a ninja in this dream and proceeded to pretend I was one. I remember having a brief hallucination of some sort during this attempt at lucid dreaming, but it was most likely from the marijuana.

After fooling around in the garage, I went inside because I was getting lonely. Frustrated with the Vow of Silence, I tried communicating with my hands and also wrote things down. The girls thought I was extremely weird, but one agreed to stargaze in the alley outback. We sat on the tailgate of my truck and looked at the sky. I wrote down for her the reasons behind the Vow of Silence, and I began to cry. I wrote how difficult a day it had been and how thinking about all the children in the world with no voice made me extremely sad. She held my hand, and I calmed down.

It was late when the girls finally left, and I decided to try to go to bed. I was restless but tired. I smoke some more pot, and it relaxed me a bit. I texted my friend Ross and bragged about my lucid dreaming experiment, and how I "figured out how to hallucinate with no drugs." This was a lie, as it was the marijuana combined with the mania that was making me see things. After texting him for a bit and telling him, I was "wicked at controlling my emotions", I finally went to sleep thinking there was another day of silence ahead of me.

23

THE LAST DAY

When I woke up the next morning, I immediately went on Twitter to continue spreading the word about my Vow of Silence campaign. I tried to get the hashtag #WEGNERISSILENT trending. I tweeted, "Enjoy my 'erratic behaviour' I'm just being myself." I followed that up with, "NOW I'M A SUPERHERO! So, enjoy my ramblings I couldn't care less whatcha think. I literally can't hear you, and my voice wasn't reaching you anyway. This is a rambly scrambly BRILLIANT TEACHER professor's Twitter account." There were no likes or retweets, but I thought I was getting my message across.

After tweeting, I saw that my old biology teacher Jared had messaged me on Twitter. He said he was thinking about me and hoped that I didn't burn myself out too fast. He told me to give him a call, which was impossible because of the Vow of Silence. My mom must have given him my number because, not long after, he texted and tried to call me.

I answered but did not speak. I quickly texted him while he was on the line, "Can't speak lost my voice." He said he understood, but I don't think he realized what he had gotten himself into – 499 texts were sent his way while he was on the line. "See that I'm not crazy yet?" "See that I'm having conversations with God?" "I'm going on a mission that's why I took a Vow of Silence." Each sentence was a separate text. I continued bragging, "I know how to manipulate and hypnotize anyone, that's why I'm silent." "It's too powerful for young Harry [Potter] to understand yet." In capital letters, I told him that the whole point of my actions was to get people to ask if I was okay (which, ironically, many did, but I turned them away). Jared, still on the line, asked if I was being bullied, and I replied, "YES I AM BEING BULLIED!"

I switched topics fast and told him that I was a writer now, then asked him randomly, "Who do you think is speaking to me when I meditate?" I never actually meditated, but when I thought I did, I was convinced that I heard the voice of God. In reality, it was merely my own voice on overdrive.

Jared was trying to explain that my actions had rattled people, especially my mother. I said, "My mother needs to be rattled." I told my old teacher that he should have been rattled more often too. I made him think that he didn't care enough about the kids in his classroom, and that he needed to be more aware. I was intentionally trying to hurt one of the nicest, kindest people around. I was on a roll. What I was saying were outright lies, and Jared had had enough of it. He started to get emotional, so he hung up the phone and began replying to me via text instead.

I was still texting in riddles and with condescension, and Jared replied flatly, "I hate riddles and condescension."

I told him that I was "rambling" and then wrote, "Everyone drinks. Wegner thinks."

Ignoring this, he asked, "Have you seen a professional?"

I told him we saw Dr Bernes two days ago and that we were scheduled to see him again in four days. I wanted to tell him more about my Vow of Silence, so I said to him that "I don't believe in time

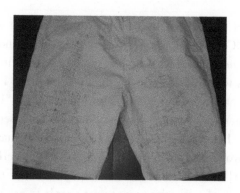

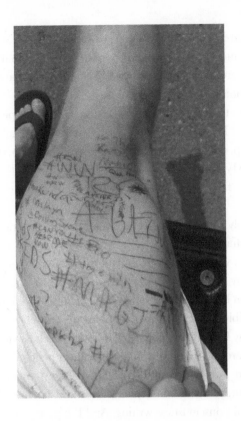

so 100 days is meaningless." I then lied and said I had "written seven articles for my blog already". Switching thoughts, I asked him if he'd invite me to go to his church, which Jared was understandably hesitant about. He received 85 texts from me before he could fit in a single reply. I told him, "Go give my mom some 'Jare Care' and tell her to stop the BIG 'Scare'."

He replied, "You need to do that yourself by approaching her where she's at. No riddles. She just needs straight talk, I think. She needs to interact on her level. That's something I think you need to trust me on."

I continued to ramble on after Jared had given me his advice, and he said, "Some of this makes sense, and some is to the point where I feel worried for your mental health. I feel like these long rants are confusing to those of us who care about you. If you don't straight up address your goals and share those specifically, you will lose people, not have them gain understanding." I continued to spam text him; finally, he said he had to take care of some errands for his family but would get back to me at some point.

I went on to leave another 90 messages on his phone; in one, I explained, "Dr Bernes said I had Asperger's so all this slow it down, shut up, don't say that, don't say this yadda yadda, drove me into sanity [sic]. My brain has been so, so confused. But that's why I talk so fast. I think… fast. Now you realize why I use my phone tactically and strategically."

Jared simply replied, "No." This ended the conversation, which had lasted more than two hours.

I realized it was now already the afternoon. I was scheduled to have lunch with my other old teacher Kevin, and I had completely blown him off. Kevin had texted me saying he waited for 15 minutes and then left. I felt terrible, so I texted him explaining my conversation with Jared. I told him how I had nearly made Jared cry, to which Kevin said, "Jason, you can't go around intentionally trying to hurt people." I spam texted him, as I had Jared, some nonsense about how I was trying to help Jared by hurting him. Kevin replied, "It's hard for me to understand your stream of consciousness writing. And I'm pretty sure hashtags are useless via text." A few more messages were sent by me until I told him, "Tell everyone I'm not crazy", and ended the conversation.

The rest of the afternoon was uneventful, and I was getting bored. I asked my friend Dylan if I could come over that night to hang out and smoke some weed, and he said sure. I texted him, "I can't wait to show you my tattoos!", referring to the writing all over myself. I hadn't showered, and was still wearing the same clothes from the previous day. I decided that it was too nice of an evening to drive, and because I had so much energy, thought it would be a perfect night for a bike ride. The sun was starting to go down when I pedalled away from my westside home toward the north side of town.

Dylan lives on the same street as my parents, which is almost 15 kilometers from my westside house. This was going to be no challenge for me, however, and I expected to have enough energy to make it back to my westside house later that night. I had my "Certainty Pack" with me, and enjoyed the ride. It was not the safest ride, however, as the route takes you down a steep hill and across a river. When I hit the hill, there was no bike path, so I was cycling on the narrow shoulder of the road, with three lanes of traffic travelling at a speed limit of 90km/h. The descent is fairly steep, and I'm not a very experienced cyclist. I was travelling pretty fast and found it hard to slow my bike down. Luckily, I didn't crash or sway into traffic. When I got to the bottom of the hill, I stopped to take a break as I was about halfway to Dylan's house. I realized what I had just done was quite dangerous. I decided to celebrate my survival with a toke of marijuana, so I sat down at a spot that overlooked some valleys.

I grabbed my one-hitter out of my backpack, as well as my headphones. I put *The Wall* on full blast through my headphones and began to sing. I stood up and began to act out the rock opera. The sun was going down and, on the side of the road, for all to see, was me with my arms flailing, dancing and shouting the words of my favourite album – I had clearly forgotten about my Vow of Silence. I did this for over an hour until it was quite dark, and I nearly lost my phone in the grass. I finally decided it was time to continue on to Dylan's place.

I entered Dylan's backyard at around 10:45pm, and I went straight to the garage to join Dylan and our friend Jordan. I wanted to show my friends that marijuana did nothing for me anymore. I packed a large bowl in Dylan's bong and smoked the whole thing in one breath. I stood up in Superman pose, then walked out to his backyard lawn to lie down. Jordan and Dylan were bewildered as they watched me roll around in the grass, high as a kite. I remember looking up at the stars, imagining I was back in Africa in my makeshift bed of chairs.

After a while, I looked at my phone, and my dad had texted me. I told him I was just down the street, but I needed space and was fine. I told him, "I have Asperger's. I've diagnosed myself… I am gonna go crazy if people keep throwing stress at me." Concerned, my dad invited me to come over when I was done at Dylan's. I agreed, and after stargazing and ignoring my friends, I said goodbye and walked down the street to my parents' place around midnight.

I was pretty tired when I got to my parents' place, but I stayed up for about another hour with my dad. We hung out in the garage and listened to a record by RUSH, a band – my dad pointed out – that completely abstains from drugs and alcohol. I reached for my medicinal marijuana from my bag when he said this, but he stopped me and offered me some of his own weed. I took a few puffs, and was soon tired enough to sleep. He said everything was going to be alright and I could sleep downstairs. Not wanting to cycle 15 kilometres home, I agreed.

My dad said he was going to sleep downstairs too, on the couch next to my bed, claiming it was too hot upstairs. Before I went to bed, I went to the washroom, and that's when I saw my reflection.

My mother has written notes of the events that happened that night. How I cycled to Dylan's, came over to their place, and freaked out after seeing my reflection. The notes say she called the mental health line at 1:30am, and they instructed her to call 911. She made the 911 call at 2am and, after arguing, I was in the ambulance by 2:45am. A new chapter in my life was about to begin, but I wasn't going into any loony bin without fighting for my freedom.

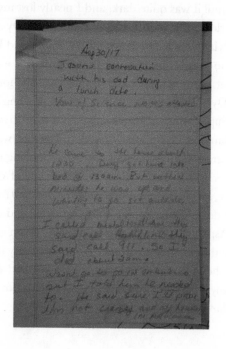

PART III

TREATMENT

24

THE HOSPITAL

After assessing me in a secluded space in the emergency room, Dr Payne made his report at 4:02am, which said he had formed his opinion on the following observations: "Jason is agitated, is talking non-stop, has written all over his arms, legs, and shorts and stated he wants to be the spokesperson for Asperger's. He does not want to stay. He shows no insight into his illness." His report then said that the following facts were communicated to him: "His parents state he is talking non-stop, he is only sleeping 3–4 hours a night. He is acting on a call from God to fix Tanzania."

Dr Payne tried to give me medicine to calm me down, but I refused. A few hours later, on 31 August 2017, I was wheeled to my "cell" in the acute psychiatry ward. My parents were with me as they wheeled me away, and they said everything was going to be alright. I was so tired, and felt dazed and confused – like that day in the United States, not long before. On the way to the acute psychiatry ward, I saw my neighbour Derrick in the lobby. He was visiting someone else, but I thought he was there to help me. I pleaded with him to rescue me as they wheeled me by; he waved hello with a concerned look on his face.

The acute psychiatry ward is an open area with rooms located round the perimeter. It has a little nook with a TV and DVD collection, a table to draw at and play games on, chairs to lounge around in, and a treadmill for exercising. The walls are white with a few basic paintings scattered throughout. The kitchen is shared with the non-acute psychiatry ward, and it's always stocked with peanut butter, crackers, fruit and other simple snacks. There is also a juice and coffee machine, but the coffee is decaffeinated, even though it says its regular.

I was taken to the "high observation" area, which has four rooms attached to it; its communal room is big and open, with a skylight so the sun can shine through. There is a shared bathroom and shower room, which does not lock. There is a security guard present at all times, and the space backs onto the nurses' station. There are several pairs of eyes on the patients at all times in this area. The rooms have windows made of unbreakable plexiglass. There are blinds in the cells, but you can only partially close them – you must be visible to the security guard at all times. The room I was given had nothing more than a mattress on the floor and a window that looked onto a brick wall and a dying garden.

My parents said goodbye and promised to visit as soon as they could. The head nurse explained my situation and handed me a pair of blue hospital pants and a yellow hospital gown to change into. Again, I was offered medication, but I refused. The nurse said it was my right to refuse

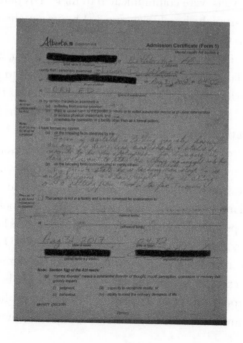

medication for one week, after which there would be an appeal hearing where I could plead my case for not taking medication. If I lost the appeal, they could legally inject the medication if I remained non-compliant. Fully alert now, I said, "I'll take everyone to court!" She handed me a "My Rights" pamphlet and the "Formal Patient" pamphlet, which explained why I was being withheld against my will, and left.

The next nurse who came in was really nice. He asked if he could get me anything, and I requested some water and a pen and paper. He returned with a blue journal and a blue pen; I told him blue was my favourite colour, and he smiled. He tried to explain to me what the medicine they were trying to give me would do for me, but I politely told him that I was not ill in the slightest and that this was all a big misunderstanding. I mentioned how I was already prescribed medicine, and asked if I could have my daily dose of it. He said under no circumstances would I receive my medicinal marijuana.

I rested and tried to get adjusted to what I called my prison cell for the rest of the day, and nothing very noteworthy occurred. The next day – the first day of September – I was bored, so I strolled out of my room to the open area. Another patient was also hanging around, so I began to talk to him. His name was Francis, and he proceeded to tell me his life story, which was fascinating. He said he was a professional gambler, with a lot of money on the outside, and he knew how to count cards. He said he had had a few brain injuries, which is why he was in the "nuthouse". He was a nice guy, so I asked him if he would like to show me the ropes of gambling sometime. He was happy to, and asked for my contact details. I said I would get a piece of paper from my notebook, but he said he'd rather inscribe it in his bar of soap – I thought this was a little off, but told him my number and mailing address nonetheless.

I was on my best behaviour for the whole day, as I wanted to appear to be whatever they thought was "normal", so I could get the hell out of there. My parents visited to see how I was adjusting, and I told them that I wanted to leave. They said I had to stay until I got better, which I said was crazy because I was already the best version of myself. The conversation was going nowhere, and they weren't allowed to stay for very long. My dad's parting request was that I take a shower and wash the ink off my body. He said my grandparents from up north wanted to visit, and that my grandfather wouldn't understand all the hashtags and quotes. I reluctantly agreed.

I took a long shower and washed the pen marks off my body. It felt good to be clean, but I did miss the reminders that I had put on my legs and arms. But, I repeated to myself, "If this is what normal is, then normal I will be." Later that night, I wrote in my journal, misquoting Pink Floyd, "I don't need no drugs to calm me. I don't need no arms around me. All in all, it was just bricks in the wall."

Because of my good behaviour, the next morning, around 7:45am, I was shown my new room, which was in the general area rather than the high observation area. The room was nice, and a definite upgrade from the cell in the high observation area. Outside the window was a beautiful lawn, and there was an actual bed, a private washroom, and even a desk with a comfy chair. My new nurse showed me around and told me that I was meeting my doctor today, Dr Palmer. I told her how I was completely sane and that this was all a mistake – I acted as normal as possible. I told her I was going to write a letter to this new doctor, and asked if she would show it to him for me; she agreed.

"Dear Mr New Doctor, Please inform Dr Palmer that he will be hearing from my lawyers (who are world-class) for withholding my legal medicinal marijuana. I do not trust this doctor. I trust my doctors. My wonderful nurses believe me… [they] are… my favourite people. Why? Because they hear me. My parents and grandparents won't even listen. I am not mad at them for they are concerned and had good intentions… Why are you telling me I have all these things when I am calm, have explained myself now over four times, yet I am still a 'formal patient'. I know Dr Palmer is a good man, and his intentions are good. My perception is he is an ignorant, quick thinking 'shrink' that won't take time to think that this 'kid' might be telling the truth. Well, sir, I hope you will hear the truth now and release me because I want to go home immediately. However, if I must 'get more rest' in the [dis]comfort of this hospital then fine. I will patiently wait like a child would. Why? Because I believe kids and I want to show them they don't need no drugs to calm them. They need a hug from a parent that won't listen. So, Dr Palmer has two options: a) he may think I am bluffing, 'delirious', 'insane', 'not fit for society' and try to rush more pills on me that I will refuse every time OR b) he may release me and 'sleep easy' knowing he doesn't have to waste his time in court because I have already begun the process of suing Dr Palmer for everything he has. Dr Payne too. Because I am not insane. You just won't hear me or listen to me. So, tick, tock, click, clock, sir. I look forward to fresh air, OR I look forward to seeing you in court. PS 'Eat My Shorts.'"

I asked the nurse to proofread it, and she laughed at the Bart Simpson "Eat my shorts" quote. She said she would photocopy the letter and show it to Dr Palmer and the head nurse. I thanked her and hung out in my room for the rest of the day until my appointment with Dr Palmer.

The meeting with Dr Palmer was short as I said, right off the bat, I wouldn't take any medicine. Dr Palmer shrugged his shoulders and said he would wait for the appeal process, and advised I get some rest until then. So, I did just that and didn't leave my room for the rest of the day. I still had a security guard watching me, who I tried chatting with a few times. His name was Ben, but he was stoic and never replied to me. He was like a statue, watching over the Manic Man that wouldn't stop talking.

The next day, I asked my nurse what my itinerary was for the day, and she wrote down that it was "to rest and relax". I tried to do this for a little while, but got really restless. I was able to get the nurse to give me some of the contents of my backpack, which was locked away in my closet. Among these was a pack of stickie notes, and I came up with the grand plan of posting the lyrics of *The Wall* on my window and wall. I wrote the lyrics on the side of the note facing the room, but on the other side I wrote messages to the outside world that I hoped someone would see and help me escape from the hospital. No one ever did, but my 39-stickie note masterpiece was completed by the time the nurse made her next round. She was taken aback at what I had done, and called in the head nurse to check it out. The head nurse wasn't overly impressed and forced me to take down what I called my "art".

She said I needed low stimulation and to rest and relax. Scribbling on stickie notes was not considered rest.

Later on in the day, my nurse informed me that I had a meeting with another doctor who would provide a second opinion to that of Dr Palmer. I tried to enter his office with my mini-Bluetooth stereo, which was also a recording device (when tethered to my phone, which was still locked away). The doctor, unfortunately, made me keep it outside the room, so I never got a chance to record his words and use them against him later, as intended.

I remember trying to tell him calmly everything that had happened over the last few weeks. I got sidetracked a few times by telling him about Tanzania, my business plans and other ideas. I just had so much information in my head, it was impossible to tell a straight story. The meeting didn't last long, and in his report the doctor wrote, "This patient is suffering from a manic episode with psychotic features. This illness leaves him without insight and unable to appreciate the illness or need for treatment." I thought I had nailed the interview, but his report was just adding to the evidence against me.

For the rest of the day, I tried conversing with the other patients, including a spy named Melody, who taught me a secret spy language; and a nice old lady who invited me to her church bake sale. I tried to convince many of the patients that the medicine they were receiving was mind-controlling and that they should stop taking it. "Look at me," I said, "I'm not taking any and I'm superhuman." Some listened, and others told me they wanted the medication. Later, the nurses asked me to stop telling patients to be non-compliant, but I just tried to be sneakier about it.

That night I was sitting alone trying to read something when a young man around my age asked if I wanted to play a game with him. More specifically, he also asked if I would "go on a date with him". I was getting quite bored, so I asked him which game he'd like to play. He said Monopoly, which is my favourite game. We sat down at the large table and played a game of SpongeBob Monopoly. I asked for his name, and he said it was Garmin; he said he knew my name was Jason. I asked how he knew my name, and it turns out that we went to the same high school. "Small world," I said. Garmin was a bit shorter than me, with tanned skin, black curly hair and awful posture. The more I thought about it, the more I recognized him. We talked for a while, and it turned out we liked similar music, movies and games. I asked him if he thought it was weird we were so similar, and he said he didn't think so. I asked him why, and he said, "It's because I am your guardian angel. I must like the same things as you." This puzzled me at first, and I asked him what the heck he meant by "guardian angel". He said he was my protector, and that he'd been protecting me all my life. He cited examples of bullies I'd experienced and the adversity I faced, and said he had helped me out in my hours of need, but sneakily. He then said that he was in the hospital now because I needed him more than ever. As he spun this tale, it made more and more sense to me. It seemed like he knew everything about me. In retrospect, he was just excellent at asking questions and then making it look like he already knew the answers, but he sure was believable.

I asked him why he was in the hospital, and he said it was because he had schizophrenia, fetal alcohol spectrum disorder (FASD) and anxiety. I didn't connect the dots at the time and see this as a connection to his wild story about being my guardian angel, but I was pretty ill myself. Garmin and I instantly became best friends, and we stayed friends for my whole tenure in the hospital. I asked him what I could do for him, being that he had done so much for me as my guardian angel, and he said that I needed to help him get free. He said that if I freed him, it would result in my own freedom. Freeing Garmin became my new main objective. Garmin said freeing him wouldn't be enough though, because he didn't really have anywhere to go after being freed. I asked him what he meant, and he told me that he had been in the foster care system for years and, because of his condition, he always needs a legal guardian even though he is legally an adult. I told him there was an easy solution: I could adopt him, and we could become brothers! He loved this idea, and we spent the rest of the night fantasizing about living together in my westside home – smoking weed (which he loved to do as well), playing games, watching movies, picking up girls for me and guys for him and, above all else, getting a puppy, which Garmin dreamed of having. We continued talking until curfew, and I saw my own history through an entirely new lens: I had had a guardian angel looking out for me the whole time.

I spent most of the next day hanging out with my new best friend. We watched movies, talked about the past, thought about the future and played more Monopoly. That night, I devised a plan to break Garmin and myself out of the hospital – I would ask the nurse to give me my phone on the pretext of finding a phone number which I wanted to call on the communal phone, but sneakily I would send out a distress signal on social media to get people to help us escape.

I executed the plan perfectly, and managed to post a tweet, tagging the organization I went to Tanzania with, Prime Minister Justin Trudeau, President Donald Trump and Tony Robbins. I was confident that one of these people would see my cry for help and free us. I briefly explained in the tweet that I was in the hospital against my will and needed help. I ended with #FREEGARMIN. Next, I went to Snapchat to tell my friends that I was okay, but as I hit send the nurse snatched my phone from me. The nurse was angry that I had lied about using my phone for accessing contact information, and said I now had to return to the high observation area. I refused, and the security guard stepped up so I could feel his presence. I reluctantly went to my old cell, waving goodbye to my guardian angel. I told him that the plan had worked, and we just had to be patient.

I wasn't tired at bedtime, but I had calmed down a bit, so figured I would stargaze under the skylight. To my dismay, when it was dark outside all you could see was reflections. I was deeply saddened I couldn't see the night sky, and longed for my nights in the open air in Tanzania. I tried to argue with my stoic security guard that it was wrong to have a skylight with no night sky; he just ignored me.

When I went to my cell, I still wasn't tired, and now that I was back in the high observation area, I didn't have much to do. I thought I would practise my public speaking, and developed a speech that I planned to deliver to world leaders one day. I was convinced that I would meet the Canadian prime minister through my old trainer, Jordie; and I also imagined meeting President Donald Trump. In this speech, which I was delivering in my cell to the imaginary audience, I laid out a plan for world peace, and then began speaking directly to President Trump. I fantasized how I would become the President's right-hand man. I even began impersonating President Trump's voice, and made up a conversation between him and myself. I must have looked completely mad, pacing my cell and talking to myself, but I was oblivious to the real people outside my room – I was in my own little world.

Talking to myself for an extended period tired me out, and I finally fell asleep. I woke up early the next morning and demanded the phone so I could call my lawyer. I didn't actually have a lawyer, but Quinn's dad was a lawyer, and I thought for sure he would fly from San Francisco and represent me, pro bono. It was now 7 September, and my appeal was on 11 September, hence the urgent need to get Quinn's dad down to the hospital as soon as possible. I called Quinn, but he didn't answer. I left a very detailed message on his phone, but he never called back. I was without a lawyer, but I felt that it would all be okay, because if I was meant to have a lawyer, I would have one – I was going to do it on my own. The trial was still a few days away, so I just tried to pass the time until then.

Still in the high observation area, I pretended that I was a Masai warrior in training. In my cell, I rolled around like a warrior would, did push-ups, and pretended I had a spear and was hunting lions. I saw a smile crack from Ben the security guard when I told him I was a Masai warrior. I told him he was like a Japanese warrior, and that I respected his stoicism very much. We got on famously after that.

When I was bored of playing pretend, I would whistle, which was my favourite pastime right then. Because I was deprived of music, I whistled songs I remembered and danced as I whistled. I was whistling so loudly that the other patients complained and I was told to stop. I was quite annoying.

Because I wasn't allowed to whistle, I asked the nurse if I could, at least, have some reading material. The nurse agreed, and I told them I had a novel in my locked-up backpack. The nurse retrieved it for me. The book was Ray Bradbury's *Fahrenheit 451*. For those that aren't familiar with the classic novel, it is a dystopian story, much like George Orwell's *1984*. Paranoia about being watched at all times and that people are out to get you are themes that course through the book. When the head nurse saw what I was reading, she immediately confiscated it. She reprimanded me, saying that I was to be in low-stimulation mode, and that I had to rest and relax. Feeling like I was in a prison, I pleaded that I was bored, but the head nurse ignored me. She said if I behaved well, I would be allowed back to the general area. I was on my best behaviour after that.

On the outside, my family was getting my affairs in order because my university courses were set to begin. They got a letter from the hospital to pass on to the university stating that I was a "formal patient" and was currently without a discharge date. I felt I had purposefully "dropped out" of university before being admitted to hospital; nonetheless, the letter meant I didn't have any withdrawals on my transcript.

After tweeting the night before, my mom had received a call from the organization I travelled to Tanzania with. They were getting in contact because they thought I was in some sort of danger and were concerned. My mom assured them I was in the hospital for a mental health issue, and that I was in a safe place and getting the help I needed. She asked them if I would have been exposed to any mind-altering substances during the trip, but they assured her that nothing of the kind would have been present. My mother was confused as to why I had come home such a different person after Tanzania; she was still trying to come to terms with my illness.

To pass the time in the high observation area, I sneakily journaled song lyrics and thoughts. I say sneakily, because I wasn't allowed my blue journal in the high observation area, because it was "too stimulating". However, I had managed to sneak in a black pocket journal that another patient had given me, as well as a pen. One song I became obsessed with was a remix of John Lennon's "Mind Games". I changed the lyrics to "Blind Games" and sang it incessantly. I was emotional sometimes when singing it because I had changed the lyrics to be about freedom. I sang and danced to this song until the nurse finally shut me up because of more complaints on the other side.

The rest of the journal was mostly more of the same manic writing I had been doing before I entered the hospital – hashtags, quotes and song lyrics. I also recorded what I thought my purpose was in life: "My purpose in life is to be the voice for the voiceless." And I created a band name for the band I planned to form when I got out; "The Society" would be three friends and me, and we would be the next Pink Floyd. I thought it was a cool name, and the idea of a band went well with my idea of writing a novel and music opera at the same time. Thinking about becoming a rock star helped pass the time until I had a visitor that afternoon.

Trevor visited me on 8 September, and it felt like he didn't stay for very long. Garmin was by my side when I sat down with him, but Trevor refused to speak to me with Garmin present. So, I told my guardian angel to sit close but to give us some privacy. I remember starting the conversation by telling Trevor that I had made him my legal guardian as I couldn't trust my parents anymore. He said he had already been informed of my decision. I don't remember much about the conversation, other than Trevor tried to explain to me that I was sick and needed treatment. He said he had researched the medication they wanted to give me and that it was okay to take. I looked at Garmin when he said this, and Garmin shook his head. I remember saying, "Not you too, Trevor," when he told me that I was sick. I still felt superhuman, and in no way did I think I had an illness. I told him I was appealing my sentence in this prison. Trevor could tell the conversation was headed nowhere; he got up to leave, and I asked him to kindly bring me some nutritious food as I didn't like the hospital food.

I didn't want to go back to the high observation area after my visit with Trevor, but the nurse said I still needed some time back there. To curb my marijuana cravings, I asked if I could have cigarette breaks, but this request was refused. However, they did offer me nicotine cartridges and nicotine gum as a substitute. I began chain-smoking these cartridges immediately; and I stockpiled my empty cartridges to show, at my appeal, how much nicotine the hospital was giving me. This strategy didn't work, however, as nobody cared how much nicotine I was having.

The nicotine wound me up a bit, and that night I was sleepless. I was on my tangent of imaginary speeches again, pacing back and forth and shouting in my room. I was annoying the nurses, and they offered me a pill to calm me down. Feeling bold, I took this pill, but I put it in my cheek and spat it out when the nurse wasn't looking. I became a master at this as I had learned how to "tongue and cheek" my medicine from Jack Nicholson in the film *One Flew Over the Cuckoo's Nest*. Nicholson played a criminal who pleads insanity to avoid going to prison and instead goes to a mental hospital. While there, he doesn't take his prescribed medication, and riles up the other patients to stop taking theirs; he causes havoc in the hospital. I truly related to this movie and character. I told my dad once when he visited that it was like I was in a sequel to the movie, which I had named, *One Flew INTO the Cuckoo's Nest*. My dad did not find this amusing.

Because I didn't take the calming medicine, I continued to be "energetic". This shift of nurses had had enough – two nurses, with two security guards, entered my cell and pinned me down. I was terrified. I was kicking and screaming to get them to let me go, to no avail. I bit one security guard as they pulled down my pants, exposing my rear end. Before I could do anything else to get them to let me go, they injected me with something that instantly made me sleepy. They laid me down gently on the mattress, and I repeated to myself over and over, "You can't do this. This isn't fair," and drifted off into a slumber that I was afraid I would never wake up from. The song "Comfortably Numb" by Pink Floyd was playing in my head as I drifted off to sleep.

The next morning, I woke up feeling rested and better than ever. I was in a good mood, relieved I was still myself after the previous night's injection. The new shift of nurses brought me my breakfast and asked if I wanted to go to the general area again. I said I did, and explained that I had had a good sleep and was feeling good. They also asked if I wanted any medicine now, but I still refused. My appeal was two days away, I explained, and I didn't want anything slowing me down.

Although I had refused my medication, the nurses handed me a printout about the medication – Quetiapine – I had been prescribed. I took the printout, underlined everything bad about the drug, and wrote in big letters "NOPE!" I looked at every possible excuse not to take the drug. I was most concerned about the part that said "call your doctor right away if you have a painful erection…[as] this may happen when not having sex… may lead to lasting sex problems, and you may not be able to have sex." I was in no way willing to give up sex for some drug I didn't need, I thought to myself.

The rest of the day I hung out with Garmin, and nothing too eventful happened. However, at night, I got into an argument via sticky note with the head night nurse about a few things I was missing. I wrote, "WHY CAN I STILL NOT HAVE HEADPHONES? Because I love music and IT calms me down [duh] and why can't I call my lawyer? Your phones don't work." In reality, their phones did work, but my "lawyer" or Quinn's dad, wasn't picking up.

In another sticky note, I wrote, "Nature's medicine is natural to humans… YOUR DRUGS made in a lab suck! MY DOCTOR SAID #MYMEDICINE HELPS ME sleep… because I have insomnia and battle with stress… so I love marijuana! So does our Prime Minister! And why do I still have a guard? My nurse said I had a great day… shift change at 11pm CHANGES EVERYTHING! Why?… How exactly AM I 'DISRUPTIVE'?" The head night nurse offered me pills to help me sleep, but I refused. The nurse appointed to me suggested I stop harassing the head night nurse or else I would get another injection. Scared of that, I sat quietly at my desk and began to read the newspaper.

The newspaper was a copy of the *Globe and Mail*. It was 1:45am when I began looking at it, and instead of reading the contents inside, I spent an hour writing all over the cover of the paper. I scribbled like a madman, and what I was writing was nonsense. I created hashtags, wrote song lyrics, posted quotes and recorded thoughts. When I was finished, I showed my nurse, and she asked if she could keep it for safekeeping in my file. I said sure, because I didn't want my new masterpiece to get wrecked. Presumably, the nurse showed this as evidence to the head nurse that I was, indeed, still manic.

The next day my parents visited. I had earlier made a wish and promise to myself that I would return to my Vow of Silence, because

I felt like no one was listening to me. I wrote in one of my journals that my one wish was "to be silent for 30 days. Why? So, I can free the children. I will only speak to #FreedomFighters because the doctors HATE MY VOICE PERIOD. My moment of silence has begun [10:05am]."

My parents arrived about an hour after this pledge, so our conversation had to be written down. My dad was agitating me because he kept trying to get me to speak. He wrote, "Sorry, I'm agitating you. Please tell me what you want me to do."

I replied, "Shut the F up AND BREATHE lol. Go to church and listen."

My mom took the pen then and wrote, "Your dad and I love and care for you, love Mom."

To this, I gave a lengthy reply. "I do too, very, very much. I do not want to hurt you or anyone. I am calm, but this doctor has misdiagnosed me, which is why I am suing them (Dr Palmer and Dr Payne). They do not want to listen to the doctors I TRUST." I then completely went off-topic and wrote, "Do you see I'm a writer yet dad? All I wanna do is act. I don't wanna sue a man for having good intentions. He is a good man, and he just doesn't understand that I legally have a prescription for legal marijuana (you know the stuff Trudeau says is good for society to consume)."

My parents left soon after I wrote that, but before they went they hugged me tight and asked if they could attend tomorrow's appeal. I nodded my head yes, and they said they'd see me the next day.

My second round of the Vow of Silence was quite successful because I mostly kept to myself. I did speak to Garmin, but only because he was a "#FreedomFighter." I spent most of the rest of the day in my room preparing for my trial. I carefully read the two pamphlets I had been given, and made notes and underlined passages that I thought would help me. The "Your Rights" pamphlet stated, "You have the right to refuse a treatment if you are mentally competent to make your own treatment decisions." Under that I wrote, "Cool, write on my file why I don't want Palmer's drugs. I want my doctor's medicine." In the "Formal Patient" pamphlet, I underlined the definition of mental disorder:

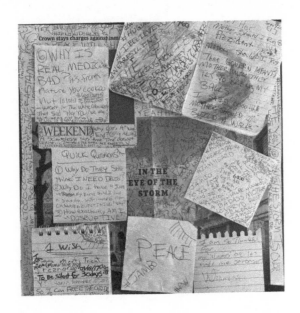

"a substantial disorder of thought, mood, perception, orientation or memory that grossly impairs; i) judgement ii) behaviour iii) capacity to recognize reality, or iv) ability to meet the ordinary demands of life." I thought having this definition to hand would be useful, because I firmly believed I in no way met the definition. However, it actually fit me perfectly. I certainly had "a substantial disorder of thought", as my mind was constantly racing; my "mood" was all over the place; and my "orientation" towards "judgement" was impaired, which affected my behaviour. I also was out of touch with "reality", in the sense that I had experienced psychosis and now believed in guardian angels. Also, when I was living on my own, I was barely meeting "the ordinary demands of life", as I wasn't eating very much, wasn't sleeping and couldn't hold down a job. I was utterly oblivious to all of these facts.

25

THE APPEAL

On 11 September 2017 at 3:45pm, my appeal trial began. I remember sitting in my room moments before, psyching myself up, thinking this was my moment for freedom and the most significant event of my life. I felt like a fighter walking to the ring when I entered the board room. The song "Thunderstruck" by AC/DC was playing in my head as I sat down, ready for battle. Thinking that my voice was the problem, I requested that I write my case down on paper. The panel, which consisted of my parents, a Board of Health member, Dr Palmer, a nurse, and a member of the community, agreed to my request. As soon as I got the purple sheet of paper, I began scribbling like the madman I was, trying to write down my life story.

I used every inch of the page, front and back and requested a second and third sheet of paper. When I had started to flip the third page to write on the back, the Board of Health member said I had to wrap it up. I wrote feverishly, pleading my case for freedom. I cited my time in Tanzania, my thriving new businesses, my hockey and school achievements, and everything I could think of that would prove I was not insane. I handed the paper in, and the panel said that they were gracious for my time and that they would get back to me later that day with their decision.

I was energized when I walked out of the room; I was confident that I had just written my ticket to freedom. I even began gathering my things in my room, because I thought I would be leaving that evening. A few hours later, as I was anxiously awaiting the decision, I was handed a sheet of paper by the nurse. I read the sheet, and my heart sank,

"The appeal for discharge has been denied. Written reasons to follow."
That was all I was given, and my nurse said that I was to start taking
my medication before bed that night. I was crushed.

The Written Reasons

The written reasons that followed days later are worth noting. The
panel does not take the act of holding someone against their will and
medicating them lightly. It was quite a process, and the panel had
to back up their reasoning. The panel documents start with some
background: "The patient is presenting manic symptoms, including
grandiosity, insomnia, overactivity and psychosis. Is in need of
hospital treatment. Family reports at least two weeks of hypomanic
symptoms." The panel documents then turn to Dr Palmer's original
assessment, which reported me as agitated, talking non-stop, lacking
insight into my illness and being obstinate in receiving treatment.
The documents cited "The Certificate of Incompetence" (dated 3
September and signed by Dr Palmer): "Patient is suffering from an
acute manic episode, refusing treatment and lacking the capacity to
decide on treatment."

The documents shone a light on the night I was admitted:
"Dr Palmer, on behalf of the hospital, stated that on August 31, 2017,

Mr Wegner came to emergency on his own will asking for help." This was a lie in my mind, but because my mom and the paramedics tricked me into walking into emergency that night, the doctors and hospital staff took it as me seeking help. The report continued, "Mr Wegner presented manic symptoms including flight of ideas... he reported poor sleep and appeared grandiose. He advised that he had been prescribed medical marijuana. Dr Palmer described Mr Wegner at the time as clearly mentally ill with a manic presentation."

The decision discussed my time in the hospital: "In hospital, he has improved a little. He remains grandiose and lacks insight. He is convinced that he can treat himself with natural means. He quotes elders from Tanzania and believes natural includes marijuana. In the hospital, he has not accepted treatment and continues to show symptoms of mania. Dr Palmer confirmed his view that there was a risk of deterioration and stated that without treatment, he felt that this risk is significant."

The nurse that was at the trial was representing the entire nursing staff, and in the next section of the documents, it said that he and the nursing staff agreed with Dr Palmer. He stated, "The manic symptoms observed by nursing include grandiose beliefs which are often tied to spirituality. Jason is refusing all medications and does not believe he needs them. He feels he can cure himself."

My parents' testimony was next; my dad advised that "the family wants the best thing for Jason's health." And my dad confirmed that "there has been a history of mood problems in the family." This statement related to my dad's youngest brother Jeff who, days after being diagnosed with bipolar disorder, ended his life. It is our family tragedy, so my situation undoubtedly spooked my family. My late uncle Jeff, like me, wanted to become a teacher, but suffered from addiction and other health issues. He was in his early thirties when he ended it all, and my family wanted to do everything possible to make sure I got the help I needed and didn't follow a similar path.

The documents concluded with the panel's reasons for its decision: "The panel accepted the evidence... that Mr Wegner suffers from a mental disorder. Symptoms have included pressured speech and grandiosity. The illness has been impairing both behaviour and judgement. The panel concluded that it is likely that the patient would suffer substantial mental deterioration if not hospitalized. The panel agreed that Mr Wegner is not willing to consider proper treatment alternatives for his mental health condition. He feels that he can treat his symptoms by natural means, including the use of medical marijuana. The decision was unanimous."

The Final Surrender

When bedtime came around, I was still in disbelief of my misfortune. I did not want to give up my superpowers, and believed that the medication would slow me down in my quest for the best life. When the nurse came to give me the medicine I was now legally required to take, I made one last act of defiance. I figured that if God or the universe truly wanted me to take the medication, they/it would give me a sign. I decided to tongue and cheek the medication, and I spat it out when I thought the nurse wasn't looking. This was a smart nurse, however, and he caught me red-handed. He said, "Okay Jason, do you want to take your medication orally for real this time or is it time for an injection?" Figuring this was the sign I was looking for, I decided to surrender and held out my hand for the oral medication. The nurse said I had to sit with him for a bit to make sure I didn't try anything else, but I assured him that I had got the sign I was looking for and was ready to begin treatment. I finally conceded that I had a mental illness, and said I was prepared to get better.

We sat and talked about the Bible for a bit, and I ate a banana with some peanut butter. I surprisingly felt okay after taking the medication, and the nurse pointed out that it wasn't all that bad. I went to bed that night with a new attitude. I was ready to accept my situation and get better. It was time to turn the page and begin a new chapter in my life again.

26

NOT AN INSTANT CURE

While I did begin taking the medication and treatment, it by no means cured me instantly. I was still in the throes of a manic episode, and my erratic behaviour continued. The following night after starting treatment, I was in my bathroom staring at the bathroom light switch, as to me it looked like a spy camera. The switch had a light underneath its cover, which I thought looked like the red recording light of a camera. I wanted to investigate whether the hospital was spying on me while I was in the washroom. Like in a spy movie, I took my mechanical pencil apart and used it as a screwdriver to loosen the bolt of the light switch cover. To my relief, there was nothing there but a miniature light bulb, and no spy camera in sight. I now became interested in the wiring, and began playing with it. I got two of the wires to spark, and it made a flame of fire. At that moment, I thought about escaping. I could start a fire, and they would have to evacuate us, and I could either run away or enjoy some fresh air for the first time in two weeks. I got out of the bathroom and started to pack up all of my things, so I'd be ready to go when the evacuation began. I didn't want to leave anything valuable in my room.

While I was packing up my room, the security guard responsible for watching me must have alerted the nurses that something was up, because moments later the head night nurse, who was not a fan of mine, caught me red-handed. She was quite upset. She said I had damaged hospital property and therefore had to go to the high observation area immediately. I asked if I could bring anything, and she responded with a firm "No". Not wanting to be bored, I demanded my Bible, which my dad had dropped off upon request a few days ago. She reluctantly agreed, and I was soon back in the high observation area with nothing but my Bible and a pen I managed to sneak in.

The security guard who was tailing me on the night shift was not nearly as cool as my Japanese warrior friend Ben. He was a short Caucasian male with Poindexter (nerd) glasses but had a nice haircut. He was not impressed with my actions, so I decided to mess with him while I was in my cell. I wasn't tired in the slightest, but I pretended to have a nap in the corner with a blanket over myself. I had my Bible in my hands, and every time the security guard tapped his foot, I matched his tap with a loud finger tap on my Bible. I found it hilarious because he looked baffled at the sound. When he got up to walk around to see if I was sleeping, I again tapped my Bible in pace with his walking step. This went on until the head night nurse came in, took my Bible away and gave me medication. This time I fully swallowed the medication and said I was done playing games.

The next morning, I woke up as energized as ever. Although I was medicated now, I was still going to bed late and waking up early. I started the morning off in my cell with a terrific speech. For some reason, my friend Chase Bell was on my mind, and I gave an impassioned speech about how I would get him to the NHL. "Chase Bell will make the NHL," I repeated. I intertwined his success on the ice with my music career. I spoke passionately, "When Bell makes the NHL, I will release my first song, and as he becomes the greatest hockey player of all time, I will become the greatest musician of all time." I felt like Tony Robbins giving a speech to thousands, pumping them up. When shift change happened and the nice morning nurse arrived, I explained that I needed my journal right away to record my thoughts. The nurse said only if I took my medication, and I said I would take it immediately as I was now fully compliant. I explained I had to get healthy so I could get out of the hospital and execute my big plans. The nurse smiled and returned with my black pocket journal.

I wrote, "CHASE BELL WILL MAKE THE NHL, AND I WILL RELEASE MY FIRST SONG WHEN HE SKATES HIS FIRST

SHIFT FOR THE PHILADELPHIA FLYERS. Till then I will sing original songs in peace. World peace will happen once I sing, but that will not happen until Chase 'Liberty' Bell makes the NHL!"

I wrote the "Massive Action Plan", which I was going to execute when I was released. First, see the Todd guy, whom I met downtown, so we could begin forming a band. Second, go to karaoke to hone my singing skills. Third, share my story. Fourth, go to school and get west of the city. Fifth, change my legal name to a cool musician's name.

I was obsessed with this goal of getting my friend to the NHL and launching my successful music career. I went to the communal space in the high observation area and began singing my favourite song that I had created, "Blind Games". I sang until I was told to stop, then whistled until I was told to stop. I sat in a chair under the skylight and imagined myself getting released on a sunny day and becoming a big success.

Around this time, Garmin came in kicking and screaming to the high observation area. He said he was coming to save me because he thought I was in danger. I told him I had already been saved and that I was very content. He just repeated his mission until the security guard and nurse closed his cell door and made him settle down. It felt like a scene from a movie, to be honest, and I felt like I was the star of my own script. I looked into Garmin's room and told him everything was going to be alright. This calmed him down, and the nurse thanked me.

I was feeling kind of tired by mid-afternoon, most likely from the medication and lack of sleep, so I lounged around in the open area and stared at the clouds like when I was on LSD, and wondered if the LSD was what put me in the hospital in the first place. I pushed that thought down because it was making me sad, and just enjoyed the sun. I remembered an article I had read in high school about "sungazing". Sungazing was supposedly a technique to replenish energy stores by staring at the sun. My biology teacher Jared thoroughly debunked this as dangerous, fake news; but, as I was tired, I thought I'd give it a try. I stared at the sun until it hurt my eyes, then I stared at the white walls of the room and thought I was hallucinating. I thought this was very cool, and did it a few more times until my eyes were sore. I didn't find any newfound energy though, which was disappointing, but it did keep me occupied enough for the nurses to agree that I was calm enough to return to the general side.

My mom visited me briefly that evening, and brought a book I'd asked for on Bobby Clarke, Chase's favourite Philadelphia Flyer. We had our first pleasant chat in weeks. She had also brought me some pizza to have for dinner, and I asked her if she could bring me some more things of comfort for the next day: "a hoody, candy, a good pen, a smile, a hug and some patience." She agreed, and we hugged goodbye.

I immediately began reading the Bobby Clarke book and making notes. I wasn't just reading the book for enjoyment, I was reading it to help with my goal of getting my friend to the NHL. I was bursting with energy and excitement imagining my friend in the NHL. I figured I would be his life coach, and decided that now would be the perfect time to start our journey. I asked the nurse for my phone to get his phone number, and promised there would be no funny business this time. I got the number (and those of a few other friends and family) in full view of the nurse, and shut the phone off – I did not want to return to the high observation area ever again.

I called Chase and, after explaining where I was and what had happened, told him all about my plans. I assured him everything was okay and that I wasn't really a prisoner anymore, and that my sights were set on freedom so I could help him make the NHL. He was pumped about my enthusiasm for his career, and I interviewed him about his hockey career at that point. He was playing junior hockey and said he wanted to make the NHL more than anything. I told him I would be his motivator, his life coach, and that the process had already begun as I had started reading the history of his favourite player.

We ended the conversation on a high note after almost an hour on the phone. It was around 10:30pm, and I decided to call another friend. Calling people became a staple in my routine over the next few weeks. The only visitors I was allowed were family, and I missed my friends. If they didn't pick up the phone, I left long and detailed messages; when they did pick up, I talked until my mouth went dry. I was still manic, but I had an attitude of recovery now. I knew I had had a manic episode, but I was confident that I would be getting out soon, and that everything was going to be alright.

In addition to my aspirations for Chase, I came up with other goals. The other "client" I wanted to have was an old hockey coach, who I knew was running a Junior B hockey club. I wanted to help him win a championship. I called him the next day and told him that I wanted to be the team's "motivational speaker" and "life coach". I neglected to tell him that I was calling him from the hospital. He was skeptical at first; to convince him, I said I would be the team's water boy to start and that all I wanted to do was be in the room with the guys. He agreed, and I was over the moon with excitement. He said he'd have to run it by the coach first, but he thought it would be great to have me on board.

Another job I gained that day was with the university radio station. I called an old regular at The Jungle who worked at the station and asked him for a position. I told him about my big ideas, and said I would start at the bottom or any available position. I explained my concept for the Wegner Ways Podcast, and starting the podcast as a radio show; I promised it would be very popular. He was thrilled to have a volunteer for the station, and said I could start learning the ropes any time. I was ecstatic.

When I told my dad about my new jobs, he wasn't impressed. He said I couldn't be making commitments in my current condition and made me call my old coach and the radio station back to rescind my applications. Both jobs are a great example of how I still wasn't better – I still had the grandiose thinking I was in some way a super being, with the ability to motivate, life coach and run a radio show with no experience.

I was also very generous around this time in the hospital. I made a list of wishes to grant, which were mostly about helping other patients gain their freedom. How I was going to do this, I still don't know. Patients have no control over other patients' fate, so I don't know why I thought I could be their saviour. I stated, in my journal, that I would free the other patients within one to three months. I also put down that I would achieve world peace in ten years, which seemed like a realistic timeline for such a goal.

Renewed Certificate

On 23 September, I got the news that I was to stay in the hospital for at least another 30 days. The renewed certificate document simply stated that I still needed hospital care and treatment, and that this was agreed upon by both Dr Palmer and the nursing staff. This upset me, and I made notes of my thoughts about their assessment all over the official documents. The documents stated that I did not want to be there, and I wrote, "Who would want to stay here?" I did, however, write that I didn't know I was bipolar, but that it made sense that I was. I ranted about how I did not come to the hospital of my own free will as it stated, and that I had been tricked. What was noticeable however is that, although I was still ranting, my writing was easier to read – my fast scribbling had slowed down, and I was becoming more logical in my writing.

Because I was upset about not being released, the nurse offered me a sheet with a lawyer's name and number. She said I could call him to see if there was anything he could do at this point. I started preparing for a call to him by making more notes and highlighting the documents, but I got tired and decided to go to bed instead. I resolved that, if they didn't think I was ready to be released, then they must know best. I didn't want to fight it anymore, and was prepared to accept my fate. I knew I was sick, and I realized that night that I still wasn't better. I had only been accepting treatment for 12 days, and the doctor and nurses had said it would take a while to see visible results. So, instead of calling the lawyer and making a big fuss about my renewal, I calmed down, took my nightly medication and retired to bed.

About a week later, I was interviewed by another doctor, Dr Rodriguez, for the purposes of updating my file. Dr Palmer was away for a few weeks, so Dr Rodriguez was to look after me. In his report, he stated, "The patient presents with a flight of ideas, pressured speech, and elevated mood. The nursing team reports... grandiose behaviours."

I remember being fond of Dr Rodriguez right off the bat. His report was accurate, but he gave me a sense of hope. We both agreed that I was ill and needed treatment, but he was the first person to paint a picture of what my life could look like when I left hospital. He said, with regular medication and a healthy lifestyle, I could still become the successful person I used to want to be. He asked what I wanted to do as a career, and I said a teacher. He said that would be an attainable career if I had the discipline to follow the long-term treatment plan and find a balance in other areas of my life. He described one of his patients who had a similar history to me – manic episode and bipolar – and went on to be a successful actor. Dr Rodriguez was the first to make me realize that my severe mental illness didn't have to limit the quality of my life. I would just have to work a little harder than someone who is "normal".

Getting Better

In the week after seeing Dr Rodriguez, I was almost a new person. I was no longer mad about my renewed admission, and had a new attitude towards getting better. My privileges were starting to increase as a result of my compliance – my parents could visit more, more food could be brought in from the outside, and I was even allowed an iPod. My dad worked out a deal with the nurses that he would control what music was on the iPod – no Pink Floyd or anything too stimulating. So, I now had one of my favourite things – music.

My dad and I were still trying to mend our relationship, which had been damaged during my weeks of mania. I was starting to reflect on my behaviour, and felt terrible about the way I had treated him. He assured me that all was forgiven, but I still felt awful. To help get us back on track, my dad created a playlist on the iPod called "Father and Son". The songs were all about the good times and tough times in father-son relationships. One of my favourite songs on the list was Cat Stevens' "Father and Son". The song particularly resonated with me when the father sings, "I was once like you are now, and I know that it's not easy / To be calm when you've found / Something going on / But take your time, think a lot / Think of everything you've got." These were very similar thoughts to what my dad was telling me at the time. He would tell me how he went through trials in his life, and at times it was hard to be calm. His advice to me was to be patient, and be thankful for what I still had and for the treatment I was getting. The song helped me see what he was saying, and it helped mend our relationship because I could see he was always looking out for my best interests.

The other song on the playlist that I really connected with was Kid Rock's "Drinking Beer with Dad." This song is about the fond memories between a father and son and the education a father instills in his son. The song made me think of all the fond memories between us, and I still get overwhelmed with feelings of love for my dad when I hear the song.

The playlist made me slow down and think about my dad and how much I loved him. I didn't want us to fight anymore. I wanted us to be like we were when I was younger. My goal was to mend my relationship with my dad and to listen to his advice, which was to focus on the endgame of my hospital stay. "What behaviours and actions are going to get you out of here the fastest?" was my dad's question to me. He said he hated seeing me in the hospital and wanted me to get healthy as fast as possible. He was unemployed at the time, having been recently laid off, so his main focus was getting me healthy and finding a new job. He visited me every day and updated my iPod every week with new music. I learned to appreciate his focus on me and cherished his daily visits.

With my dad helping me stay focussed in the hospital, I was starting to improve. The doctor removed my 24/7 security guard, and I was even allowed to go outside, supervised, once a day for 30 minutes. My mom took me on my first walk outside, and the breath of fresh air was the greatest thing in the world. I still had an elevated mood, however, and when we were walking, I tried to talk to a few strangers on the street, but my mom ushered me away from them. She said I had to remember society's norms and behaviours if I ever wanted to get out of the hospital. After that, I tried to re-centre myself and recall what "normal" was.

In addition to gaining outside privileges, I was moved to a shared room, where I stayed for the remainder of my time in the hospital. My first roommate was an older gentleman who identified as a Catholic.

I was on a bit of a religious kick, and called myself a Christian. He became really impressed with me, and eventually thought I was the second coming of Jesus. This fed into my ego, and for a few days, I too thought I was Jesus. I even told my roommate that a big storm that was happening in the United States was because I was having a bad day, and God was angry at the world for giving me a bad day. He believed this, and my charade as Jesus continued.

After a couple of weeks, by which time I had come to my senses and realized I was not Jesus and that storms didn't happen because I had a bad day, I got a new roommate. He was a middle-aged man, and was the most sane person I met in the hospital. He was suffering from a bout with post-traumatic stress disorder (PTSD), and our conversations were quite normal. We got along really well, as we were both ice hockey fans and supported the Edmonton Oilers. He helped me stay grounded, and I think having him as a roommate helped my recovery.

While I didn't think I was Jesus anymore, I did think, for a while, that I had met God in the form of a senior patient named Barry. He never spoke – he only ever smiled or mumbled. I began treating Barry like a king. I would sit and talk with him about life, and I regularly gave him my dessert at dinner as a tithing.

About a week into October, Dr Palmer gave me the privilege of "home visits". This meant that I could go home to my parents' place for three hours and do whatever I wanted under their supervision. I was ecstatic, but my first visit home was almost too much. Being out of society for almost six weeks and coming down from a manic episode was a lot for my body and mind to take. When I got home, the scenery was almost overwhelming because I was so used to the blankness of hospital. But this was the purpose of the home visits: to help me reintegrate. I remember being a bit angry that they had moved me out of my westside home and that all my stuff was back at my parents' place. However, they and Dr Palmer agreed that it would be best for my recovery if I lived at home, at least for a while. I got over it pretty fast, and tried to soak up my three-hour break from the hospital.

I remember my parents telling me to slow down and enjoy my home visit, but I just wanted to do everything. I tried listening to music, plugging in a movie and playing video games. I couldn't pick an activity, so I decided to do everything, and before I knew it, it was time to go back. The visit was a taste of freedom, and it made me even more determined to recover and get out of the hospital as fast as possible.

On a subsequent home visit, my parents allowed a few of my friends to visit. I remember still being a little erratic – I showed them my new stereo and how powerful it was; and I remember telling them that, although I was medicated, I still thought I was seeing things. I jumped up on a bar stool, held my phone up with its flashlight on and shone it on the TV. I explained to them I was seeing colours in the reflection of the TV, and it was the same colourful hallucination I experienced when I was on LSD. My friends laughed and said that everybody saw those colours, and that it was perfectly normal. This made me feel better.

Back in the hospital, my journal reflects the new attitude I was exuding. No longer was I hyper-energized, obstinate and pushy. The medication had calmed me down immensely, and I had re-centered myself. In one journal entry, I wrote down 33 things I was grateful for, such as, "My dad who does everything possible to help me recover, my mother for sending me to get the help I need, my sister, my grandparents, my doctors and nurses who are helping me through my recovery and myself for not giving up and avoiding temptations." It shows my change in attitude, particularly towards the hospital staff.

In another entry, I wrote down a revised version of "My Purpose in Life". I wrote that my purpose is to "live, give and be the soul that helps the helpless. I wanna be the teacher that gets through to the kids no one wants and then be the teacher that teaches teachers how to do what I can do, which is to reach the unreachable. It is my gift in life, and I am so, so grateful. I am grateful for this pain and for this 'invisible illness' because I am a fighter and I will win."

I was starting to get optimistic by the end of my stay and was confident that the entire ordeal was merely a setback. This entry was the first time I had expressed confidence in overcoming the "invisible illness", and also shows my aspirations for being a teacher again.

I was starting to show strong signs of recovery in mid-October, and because I was calm and collected, the nursing staff allowed me to start participating in activities that the other patients were doing; this included group talk therapy and recreational therapy. In group therapy, we would sit in a circle and discuss various issues and problems with having a mental illness. We did different activities to springboard conversations, but it was basically talking therapy as a group. I really enjoyed the discussions, and always offered to speak when it was my turn. I wanted to help other people in their recovery too, so I always offered my perspective or quoted Tony Robbins. The only time I felt uncomfortable at the group therapy was when there was a Satanist present. He was a mean fellow and shot down everything anybody said. He was extraordinarily pessimistic and rude. I tried to reason with him and show him that life wasn't so grim, but he challenged everything I said and made me feel bad. The nurses soon stopped him attending because he was sucking the energy out of the room. I kept my distance from him for the rest of my stay in the hospital. I'm not sure if he ever got the help he needed, but I hope he has a better outlook on life now.

Recreational therapy was an absolute treat – it was a break from everything else and a chance to play games and eat popcorn with two wonderful, nice women from the nursing staff. When it was time for recreational therapy, we would go to the games room and either play billiards or foosball. It was always a blast, and the other patients loved it too. We could also choose to do art or kick back and relax and forget about being in the hospital. It certainly lifted my spirits while I was in the hospital, and I think it was integral to my recovery as a whole, because it made me remember that life could still be fun.

When I was nearing my last days in the hospital, I started to reflect on my behaviours during my episode. It was clear to me that I had treated some people poorly, and that I had relationships to mend. One of those relationships was with my old teacher Kevin. While on a home visit, I messaged him on Twitter; I apologized for the way I had treated him and told him I was getting better. His response was encouraging: "You have a tremendous potential to be a positive influence on people, and I am certain that the past weeks will only serve to strengthen your story." This comment made me think about my story and realize that it was by no means over because of this setback. It was merely another chapter in the big scheme of things.

Discharge

On 25 October 2017, I was discharged from the hospital. I had been looking forward to this day for weeks, and I felt more than ready. I was reasonably adjusted to the medication – in the sense that I was no longer in mania – and I was sick of being in the hospital. I was confident that I was ready for the challenges that lay ahead in the real world. The hospital staff parted ways with me by giving me a "Discharge Care Plan". It said I was to "bath or shower daily, eat nutritious meals and snacks, and participate in physical activity as tolerated." It then listed the three medications I was taking, provided an address for an Intro to Recovery and Living Sober group therapy session and, lastly, in capital letters, it said, "ABSTAIN FROM DRUGS/ALCOHOL." These were also the parting words from the head nurse, and she made me promise never to do marijuana again. I agreed, knowing full well that it would send me right back to the hospital, which is a place I never wish to return to.

My mom was the one to take me home that day as my dad was training for his new job. When we got home, I was quite tired from saying my goodbyes and realizing that I was free. It felt like I had just gotten back from a long journey . My mom suggested that I take it easy and watch a movie, so I did just that. My new reality and the next phase in my life was just beginning, and it would also be a long journey.

PART IV

RECOVERY

27

LIVING WITH BIPOLAR I DISORDER

In one of my pocket journals, I wrote, "My job is to do what will make me balanced." This was my aim when I got out of the hospital. I had regained my freedom, but I wasn't right just yet. I had moved back home, but it felt strange; the way my mom had organized my room was slightly different than when I had packed up and left. I was still shy of my reflection to an extent, and asked my mom if we could take down the big mirror in my room. She said she didn't think that was a good idea, but offered to help me redecorate my room the way I wanted. We did just that, and I then felt a lot more comfortable at home and began to accept that I needed to live with my parents.

My early days were filled with a lot of rest, as I was only supposed to do two things in a day. For example, "Go to therapy and do yoga," or "Go for a walk and watch a movie." Low stimulation is what the hospital had prescribed, and I was adamant about following orders now.

The therapy I was attending, in the beginning, was a Living Sober group offered through mental health services. Over three weeks, a psychologist taught the group about the brain and how addictions work. The sessions were four times a week for three hours a day. I was the only bipolar person there, and I was quite shy and tired. It was a complete juxtaposition to my days in the university classroom, where I was energetic and always raised my hand. The class was somewhat helpful in reintegrating me into society, and the psychologist was phenomenal, but I wasn't really in a state to learn yet, so I stopped attending after about a week.

One thing I did take away from the group was a booklet explaining what bipolar disorder was and how to recover from it. I read this carefully, as I wanted to learn everything I could about my condition. It starts by saying that you should "learn to live with rather than suffer from [your disorder]." It noted that recovery "takes time, patience and courage", and that, "with proper treatment, it is possible for many people with bipolar disorder to function well." I found this very encouraging, and as a reminder of this, I wrote "Patience" on a sticky note and posted it in my room. It's still there, and it was the virtue I had to remind myself of constantly throughout my recovery.

I was interested to learn that "bipolar disorder affects approximately one out of every 100 people". Their description of mania was spot on as well: "In the manic period... you feel superhuman. Your thoughts and ideas are radically ambitious. Less need for sleep... [and] pressure to keep talking. You speak quickly and can't stop talking... ideas or thoughts race through your mind." Now that I was getting better and understood I had bipolar disorder, I could see how well this description fitted me.

I found what the booklet said about drugs encouraging: "Using drugs doesn't cause bipolar disorder, but these events can create stress that may trigger or affect the course of the illness." For a while, I blamed myself for causing the episode because of my experimentation with LSD. I have since learned that, while the LSD certainly did not help matters, it was not a direct cause of the episode. That being said, psychedelic drugs and any other mind-altering drugs, such as marijuana, are completely untouchable for the bipolar person that wants to get healthy, as it can be a trigger for another manic episode.

Another encouraging thing I learned from the booklet was that I was doing well now because I had received treatment. It said, "If bipolar disorder is not treated, people tend to have longer, more frequent episodes. They generally have chaotic lives and many problems with little hope of things getting better." After reading that, I was determined that that would not be me. One episode was enough.

The booklet ended by saying not to lose hope, as "people with bipolar disorder can have satisfying and productive lives." However, it did say that you must "recognize that stigma exists" and "navigating that stigma can be challenging." I kept both of these things in mind throughout my year of recovery, and tried to remember that things do get better as time passes.

Meeting the Doctors

My first meeting with Dr Palmer outside the hospital environment was productive. We started our long journey of medication tinkering, as I described to him that things didn't feel quite right. We adjusted the doses of the three medicines and went from there. Dr Palmer said that my recovery would take about 10 to 18 months, and that I must remain patient and follow the plan laid out for me. He preached that family support, healthy lifestyle and a low-stress life was critical for my recovery. He scheduled me to check in with him regularly, and I saw Dr Palmer every two to four weeks for a year, until we got the medication right.

About ten days after getting out of the hospital, I had my second session with my psychologist, Dr Bernes. We touched bases, and the session was much different to the first one. There was no secret recording or long rambles; it was just a thoughtful conversation. My mother came too, and went on to attend all of my sessions with both doctors, as a second voice to add to the discussions. She would also issue reminders to me when we left the office. This second session with Dr Bernes was helpful, and we had appointments every three to four weeks over the next year. As beneficial as these appointments were, I couldn't avoid the inevitable, which was a bout of depression. What goes up must come down, and because I was on such an up when manic, I was destined for a downwards turn.

Meeting the Doctors

28

DEPRESSION

For those who have experienced depression, I am sure they will agree that it is hard to describe how it feels to someone who has never experienced it. For me, it was a constant state of dullness and tiredness. A lot of the time, I didn't want to do anything; I remember constantly telling my mother this. I just wanted to lie down and stare at the wall. At least I didn't get the feelings of worthlessness that some who have suffered depression describe – perhaps because I understood that it was part of the recovery process. It was incredibly unenjoyable, nonetheless. I would say my bout with depression lasted at least seven months, from October 2017 to May 2018. It was a challenging time.

During my depression, I remember going for a winter walk with my dad. I was feeling quite crummy, and was reflecting on my behaviour during my episode. I told my dad that I was sorry for how I had treated him and what I had put the family through. He said that he had forgiven me a long time ago, and knew that I couldn't control my behaviour at that point. He said that he blamed himself for the episode, because he thought he had passed the bipolar genes to me. I assured him that I placed no blame on anybody, especially not him, and that he should drop that theory altogether. Being bipolar was nobody's fault. It was just something that happened to me, and was out of anybody's control. It felt good for both of us to get these thoughts off our chests, and our relationship after that walk only grew stronger as the days passed.

Something I tried to help me through my depression and make sense of my disorder was religion. I started attending church with my dad regularly in the fall I was discharged. A few times it helped, but altogether I decided it wasn't for me. I wasn't brought up in a particularly religious household, and my beliefs before my episode were agnostic. After attending church for a while, I went back to that way of thinking, and that's what I believe to this day. I respect all religions and can see the good they bring out in people. Personally, I operate better as an agnostic rather than being part of one religion.

Back to Work

Being depressed was making me restless, and I missed working. I was not ready to go back to work by any means, but I attempted to get my jobs back nonetheless. I went to my bar manager at The Jungle first and asked him for my job back. He said that although my actions were out of my control, the misdemeanours were still too serious to let me come back. I had damaged the reputation of the bar on the night of the wedding, and the owner of the bar said I was not to come back under any circumstance. I was quite disappointed, but I figured I would definitely get my job back with the catering company.

To my dismay, the catering company said they had replaced me. It was down season for them, and they simply didn't need me. They said I could check back with them in the spring, but I never did. It seemed that, perhaps, they didn't want me back, and I never wanted to be somewhere I wasn't wanted.

Before finding a new job, I tried volunteering at the local food bank for a while. My shifts were only two to four hours long, but that was long enough. It was tiring but rewarding work, and it made me feel better some days. I worked for about a month during the winter season, and I gradually felt like I was ready to take on a real job again.

In the spring, I applied for a bartending job at a local pub called The Beehive. I didn't crush the interview by any means – I was shy, tired-looking and lacking confidence. I remember being exhausted after the ten-minute interview, but I got the job anyway as they were desperate. My first shift was eight hours long, and I barely made it. It was mostly training and refreshers on how to bartend, which was fine, but the length of time standing was excruciating. I just didn't have the endurance to last a full shift. I was scheduled to work the next day, which would have been St Patrick's Day, but I quit before the shift started. I was so drained after one eight-hour shift that I knew I wouldn't make it through a busy shift like St Patrick's Day. I was so ashamed of having to quit that I had my dad phone the manager to explain that I was recovering from a manic episode and that I was depressed. The manager understood, and there were no problems, but it still made me feel bad.

It's important to note that during my depression, every time I did something for the first time, I became exhausted. The first time I got together with friends, or the first session of church, and definitely that first shift of work, were absolutely draining. It got better every time I did something twice, but it was certainly tiring trying to do anything for the first time after coming out of hospital.

Side Effects

Throughout depression, we tinkered with my medication a lot, and some side effects are worth noting. The most drastic side effect was weight gain. When I entered the hospital in late August 2017, I was a skinny 175lbs. My highest recorded weight a year and a half later was 252lbs. This drastic weight gain left my body with stretch marks.

Another side effect I had for a while was a chattering jaw and shaky hands. I didn't last long on the mixture of medication that was causing this because it was affecting my lifestyle.

Lastly, the other side effect I experienced was emotional bluntness, which felt like an extension of depression – I felt nothing all the time. I was even-keeled all day long, every day – I was neither happy nor sad, just neutral. It was a boring way to live, so I didn't last long on that cocktail either.

Adjusting your medication is normal for anyone trying to recover from a manic episode. Everyone's body is different and reacts to the medication differently. I came to this realization when I made friends with an old co-worker from The Jungle, Cliff, who is also bipolar. Cliff helped me immensely throughout my year of recovery, as he had been through it all before. He is a few years older than me and has had three manic episodes. The last two were both, he thinks, triggered by marijuana use, and he warned me never to use marijuana again. He said a manic episode is like having a heart attack on the brain, and that each episode causes some brain damage, according to his doctor. Hearing his story was helpful, because he is living proof that it does get better, and that you can function in life with bipolar disorder. He has now graduated from university, and we remain friends.

Back to School

While I still wasn't feeling 100 per cent better, the doctors and I agreed that by January 2018, I was well enough to return to school. I had become bored out of my mind sitting around all winter, so I was excited to try school again. I knew it would be hard, but I figured it was time to try a light load of classes. I signed up for three classes, and Dr Bernes encouraged me to take three interesting classes. I wanted the classes to work toward my degree, so I somewhat ignored him. The result was nearly disastrous.

I picked a business ethics course, a marketing course and a sports marketing course. I lasted a day in the sports marketing class before swapping it for an introductory sociology course. My mixture of classes was unenjoyable, to say the least. I was still depressed, so I was almost always tired when I went to school, and the material was so boring that I barely made it through. The sociology course was alright, and I got an A- in it, which was good, but the business ethics and marketing courses were two of the worst university classes I have ever taken. The content was dull and poorly delivered by the professors. The reading lists were also dry, and it was hard to do well in the courses. The business ethics course required a presentation, however, which was good exposure for me, as I hadn't spoken in front of a crowd for a long time. I did fine, but I sure was nervous.

I didn't excel in either of the courses, getting Bs in both. It wasn't a fun semester, and I began to question if I was in the right field. I discussed it with Dr Bernes, and we concluded that I should give English another try. I resolved that I shouldn't let one person (the teacher mentor from my first round of Education 1000) decide my path in life. I had always been passionate about English, and I enjoyed it. I changed my degree back to an English major before the semester was over, and luckily my year and a half of business classes transferred into a minor, so no time was wasted in the big scheme of things.

The semester ended with me still in a depression, and I was getting sick of feeling low and tired. The med tinkering didn't seem like it was going to be enough to get me out of my depression, and I expressed this to Dr Bernes. He and I had been doing a few things to try and combat the depression, but we both decided I needed a holistic approach to recovery. What we came up with together was life-changing and got me out of my depression – we call it "The Octagon of Life".

29

THE OCTAGON OF LIFE

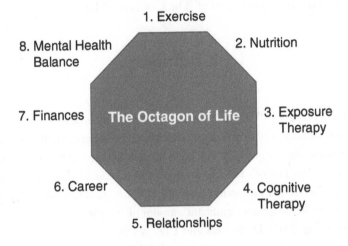

1. Exercise

8. Mental Health Balance

2. Nutrition

7. Finances

The Octagon of Life

3. Exposure Therapy

6. Career

4. Cognitive Therapy

5. Relationships

1. Exercise

The first thing Dr Bernes told me to do when I got out of the hospital was to start exercising. As I was coming down from a major manic episode, the strategy was to start small and gradually build up my minutes and intensity of exercise. I started by taking 20-minute walks four or five times a week, and then I built it up to about 20 minutes of strength training four or five times a week instead of the walks. The goal was to be able to complete an hour of high-intensity exercise.

Luckily, I had a terrific trainer in Trevor, so I had great strength training programmes.

Over a year, I gradually built myself up to consistently complete at least three one-hour workouts of 45 minutes of strength training and 10 minutes of high-intensity intervals. Getting to the gym was not easy to begin with, as during my depression it was tough to motivate myself to leave the house. However, because it was gradual, once I got the medication balance right, I was able to go to the gym consistently. Consistently doing three workouts a week for several months resulted in significant changes. However, these changes would all be for nothing if it weren't for the next part of The Octagon of Life.

2. Nutrition

As the saying goes, "You can't outrun a bad diet." This could not be truer. Immediately after setting me up with an exercise regime, Dr Bernes and I discussed my eating habits. I have been a healthy eater since being introduced to Trevor's HARD Training when I was 14. However, when I was depressed, I ate poorly, and some of the medications, as I have noted, made me gain a significant amount of weight.

In spring 2019, Dr Bernes and I really honed in on nutrition, and created a nutrition and lifestyle plan. I did my research before coming to Dr Bernes with the idea of changing my diet, and I started by going to the person with the most expertise I knew, Justin Kanigan. Justin was my trainer at HARD Training when I was a kid, and he's now a health coach and traditional Chinese medicine practitioner. He's also incredibly fit and one of the healthiest guys I know. Justin advised that I look into the low-carb, high-fat diet, as well as intermittent fasting. The importance, Dr Bernes stressed, was to find a nutrition plan that would work for me and my lifestyle. The low-carb, high-fat diet, combined with intermittent fasting, produced phenomenal results. After nine months of my nutrition plan, I had lost 70lbs! However, it is important to note that the results would not have been as drastic if the diet hadn't been combined with high-quality exercise.

3. Exposure Therapy

My manic episode was, in many ways, traumatic. To combat the trauma I had experienced, Dr Bernes and I targeted the emotional baggage I was carrying. When I got out of hospital, every thought I had about my manic episode made me feel extremely low, and every time I was reminded of my manic episode, I felt ashamed of who I had become. To treat my shame and overcome these insidious thoughts about my manic episode, Dr Bernes recommended that I do exposure therapy.

Dr Bernes is an expert in exposure therapy, which is basically facing one's trauma head-on in a controlled environment. Dr Bernes works with the local Royal Canadian Mounted Police (RCMP) regularly, and post-traumatic stress disorder (PTSD) is a common issue. To combat PTSD, Dr Bernes has the RCMP officers engage in exposure therapy immediately following a traumatic event. For example, Dr Bernes explained to me how one RCMP officer he had worked with had faced a traumatic event at a scene of a crime – he fired his weapon at someone. Following this, the officer couldn't pass the crime scene without breaking down and shaking uncontrollably. Dr Bernes told him to immediately drive to the crime scene and face his emotions head-on. Crying, shaking and being angry was all encouraged. The goal was to flood himself with the emotions that were bottled up and release them, so they didn't hold him back anymore. After engaging in exposure therapy, the officer was able to take back control of his life and continues to be a successful RCMP officer.

In extreme cases, Dr Bernes will have his clients build up their exposure therapy, starting with 15-minute sessions and working up to an hour of intense emotion. The goal is to do exposure therapy as many times as it takes until one has a neutral or better feeling about the situation. Dr Bernes argues that exposure therapy is effective for treating all types of trauma and can be done by anyone.

I did my first round of exposure therapy immediately after Dr Bernes explained it to me. This involved starting to reading over my journals, listening to my audio recordings, watching the videos I had posted to social media, and thinking about my episode in its entirety. I thought about the drugs I had taken and the consequences of them. I reminded myself of the jobs I had lost and the people I had hurt. I listened to myself ranting on the streets. I also reminded myself of the money I had wasted and the time I had lost from being in the hospital. I flooded myself with every negative emotion and thought I could remember from my episode for an hour a day until it didn't bother me anymore. This process was hard and emotionally terrifying, but because I did it in a controlled way, it was safe to do. In all, it took about ten days before I was feeling neutral about the events of my manic episode and, as the days went on, I gradually felt better, and could even see some of the humour in them. I also realized that I had survived my manic episode, and that it was now just a chapter in my life.

Right around the time when I had completed my exposure therapy and was feeling better about my manic episode, my friend Sydney approached me for a mental health project she was working on. It was called Seeing Mental Illness, and she thought I would be perfect for the project. Seeing Mental Illness is a photography project that aims to show everyday people who live with a mental illness but are not limited by it. For the project, she took two pictures of each participant, one in black and white illustrating the mental illness, and the other in colour, illustrating the participant living a normal life. For my black and white photo, I posed looking distressed and disheveled with one of my manic writings in view. The second photo was a bright picture of me walking my dog. I also wrote a description of my episode, and how I was recovering from and living with a severe mental illness.

Sydney posted the story on both Facebook and Instagram under the handle "@seeingmentalillness", and mine was the first story. The response and support was phenomenal. A couple of hundred people saw and liked the post, and dozens of people commented on my story, issuing words of encouragement. It felt great to finally get my story out there, and to come out as a bipolar person who isn't limited by their illness.

Of course, the most significant exposure therapy I have done is preparing and writing this book. At times, it has been emotionally draining, especially listening to the audio journals, but I feel comfortable with my story now. I owe that to Dr Bernes' exposure Therapy. Without exposure therapy, the baggage I was carrying would have continued to creep into my life and weigh me down.

4. Cognitive Therapy

It is tough to motivate yourself to stick to a nutrition and exercise regime if you continuously have limiting thoughts such as, "I'm no good", or "This will never get better". I was struggling with negative thoughts, even after completing my rounds of exposure therapy. What I was suffering from is known as "cognitive distortions". To combat my cognitive distortions, Dr Bernes got me to engage with cognitive therapy. This is the act of consciously challenging your limiting beliefs, or cognitive distortions, and replacing them with better, more rational thoughts. The way Dr Bernes described cognitive therapy was by using the ABCDE model.

A – Event
B – Cognitive Distortion
C – Bad Feeling
D – Disputing Cognitive Distortion
E – New Feeling

A (the event) causes B (cognitive distortion), which results in C (undesirable feeling). Cognitive therapy takes place in D (one disputes the cognitive distortion), which results in E (a better feeling).

I needed to learn to use cognitive therapy because I had some limiting beliefs about myself and my illness. For example, I couldn't stop feeling crummy after hanging out with my friends when they would use marijuana and drink alcohol. It made me feel bad that I couldn't get in on the "fun", and that I would never have any friends again. I had to dispute these thoughts if I ever wanted to feel better. So, I had to think about and write out the reasons why my feelings or cognitive distortions were wrong. Using the ABCDE model of cognitive therapy, my situation looked like this:

A – Being around friends that are using substances

B – "I'm worthless", "My life sucks", "I'll never be able to socialize"

C – Feeling worthless

D – "Do I really need substances to have a good life?" "Don't I enjoy other things?" "Can't I still socialize with a water in my hand?"

E – Feeling better about the situation, and not bummed out every time I hang with my friend.

With Dr Bernes' cognitive therapy technique, I was able to begin hanging out with friends and overcome my cognitive distortions.

5. Relationships

Dr Bernes told me that a bad relationship can affect all the areas of my life that are meaningful. It can cause binge eating, and create emotional baggage and limiting thoughts. Therefore, finding a high-quality relationship with the right person became the next area of focus for my recovery. To achieve this, Dr Bernes had me create what he calls "relationship criteria". Essentially, relationship criteria is a detailed description of what the perfect partner would be. Dr Bernes told me that he believes there is more than one soulmate out there for me, but that it was important I create my relationship criteria before I enter "the field", because if I wasn't clear on what I wanted, I would be never be able to find a great match.

Dr Bernes told me that the relationship criteria is about more than just looks. I needed to list the ideal personality, character traits, behaviours and common interests I wanted in the perfect partner. Dr Bernes stressed that I be as detailed as possible, which resulted in me listing over 70 items in my relationship criteria. Some of the items on my list were: smart, money-conscious, easy to talk to, down to earth, humble, great hair, and likes music similar to me. He said this level of detail was great, and that I would now be hyper-aware of when a person meeting that criteria walked into my life.

After creating my relationship criteria, I met a woman named Emma, who was very good-looking. At first, she seemed like she matched my criteria, but after about three weeks, I came to my senses and realized she was only hitting 65 per cent of it. She wasn't a very good person once I really got to know her, and we certainly didn't see eye to eye on a lot of issues. I luckily got out of the relationship before I was too deeply invested. Afterwards, I went back to my relationship criteria and readjusted it. Dr Bernes said that readjusting the relationship criteria is an important thing to do, and it should be looked at as an ongoing and developing document.

With dating, Dr Bernes told me that I should be able to tell if a person is hitting my criteria by the third meeting. He said that by the third meeting I should have gathered enough information to determine if a relationship with this person is worth pursuing. After some practice, I was able to determine if a woman would be a good fit within one 45-minute coffee meeting. I did this by developing what I like to call "Criteria Questions". The questions aim to direct the conversation to topics that are related to my criteria. For example, I like to ask what they are studying or what their perfect job would be. Another typical question I ask is, "What do you like to spend your money on?" and, "Are you a night in or a night out type of person?" Questions like these help me determine if the girl is smart, money-conscious and if they like to party (which I do not).

Dr Bernes concluded our discussion on relationships by saying that the indicator of a good match was determined by the following three things. First, does it feel like you're seeing your best friend? Second, is there a feeling of intense attraction? And, last of all, can you show up every day for this person and be there for them? If you can answer "yes" to these three questions, then you may very well have hit the jackpot and found a partner worth sticking with.

6. Career

The sixth area of The Octagon of Life had to do with my future. Dr Bernes explained that many people are dissatisfied with their job, which affects other areas of their life. Being unhappy at work can cause a person to stress eat and gain weight, can produce limiting thoughts and affect the meaningful relationships in their life. As I, like everyone, will spend a good majority of my life in the workforce, it is vital for my wellbeing and fulfilment to find an occupation that I enjoy. His advice was to do what I loved. He explained that people who love their job are happier, healthier and live better lives.

When I was trying to decide what career I wanted, I asked the question: Who are the happiest people I know? My answer was teachers, and I wanted to be like them. I had developed a love for English and education studies long before I met Dr Bernes, so we established that this would be the career worth pursuing and focussing on for me.

Dr Bernes suggested that if I had been struggling to figure out what occupation would fulfill me the most, I could have taken the idea of relationship criteria and extended it to career criteria. He said you just need to make a list of all the things you want in the ideal job, such as: helps others, is challenging, not too stressful, enjoyable, etc. He said that if you only look for a job that pays well, but is unenjoyable, it would affect the other areas of The Octagon of Life and therefore recovery. I reassured him that I was satisfied with my choice and that I may even consider pursuing a PhD in education one day. He said this was a great idea and that there was no ceiling on my potential.

The result of our conversation on careers was a solid career plan that gave me a peace of mind in my day-to-day activities. We were clear on the type of classes I needed to take to become a teacher, and the possible steps I would need to take towards becoming a professor. I also researched the typical salaries and benefits that teachers and professors get so I could plan out my financial future. Creating this career plan was integral to combating my depression.

7. Finances

The seventh area of The Octagon of Life that Dr Bernes focussed on with me was finances. Money was something I had always been good with before my manic episode. During my manic episode, however, I spent money recklessly and had virtually no streams of income. Prior to my manic episode, I was great at saving more than I spent, and at spending wisely. Trevor had told me when I was 15, "Money won't bring you happiness, but the absence of money will undoubtedly bring you stress and pain in your life," which sparked an interest in money and investing from then on. Dr Bernes wanted to reignite my passion for finances and develop a plan for wealth and financial freedom.

He began the discussion with saving. He suggested that, because I lived at home and my expenses were low, I start saving at least 50 per cent of every paycheck I earned. I upped his challenge to 60 per cent, and began regularly saving that much of whatever I earned to replenish my bank accounts. Dr Bernes stressed that I would not be able to earn my way to financial freedom by my paycheck alone, which is why he suggested I put some money aside for investing.

However, before I invested any money, he wanted to ensure I had taken care of any debt I had. I cleared the credit card debts that had accrued due to all the incompetent purchases I made during my episode. Thankfully, I did not have any student loans or debt of that kind because my grandparents from up north have kindly paid for my education.

After my debts were taken care of, Dr Bernes made sure I had a Registered Retirement Savings Plan (a pension) in place and a tax-free savings account open. This was to ensure I had accounts that I could put investments in and have them tax-sheltered. Then Dr Bernes instructed me to put a percentage of my income in a regular savings account, so that I would have easy access to money if I ever needed it.

Next, Dr Bernes explained a future strategy for when I moved out of my parents' place.

He recommended that I look into real estate and start thinking about and researching buying a house. The discussion on real estate was an extended one, as Dr Bernes instructed me to look at everything from house prices, square footage and neighbourhood demographics. He wanted me to develop what he called a "design eye", or an eye for detail, when it comes to houses. We discussed the process of buying a house, and he said that it was not out of the realm of possibilities for me to buy a starter home and pay it off within five years. He said that with my savings plan and the possibility of renting out a portion of the house, I could easily accomplish this ambitious goal of paying off a house in five years.

Dr Bernes continued the discussion of real estate with his thoughts on a second house, or more specifically the "dream home". He said that if I was to pay off the first house fast, continue to save like crazy and rent out most of the house, I would be able to save towards moving into my dream home. Once moved in, I could continue to rent out the first house to help pay for the second house. It was all a brilliant plan, and got me very excited about my financial future.

Once we were finished discussing bank accounts and real estate, Dr Bernes stressed that it was also important, financially, to maximize whatever benefits I was receiving. Because my mother is a school district employee, I, as a student, receive pretty good benefits. That being said, I realized I had not been maximizing them, so after our discussion I began booking more chiropractic appointments and massages so that I could realize the full potential of the benefits I was on.

The final thing Dr Bernes and I discussed in regard to my finances was the stock market. The stock market was something I was familiar with (I had bought some marijuana stocks with the company that fulfilled my medicinal marijuana prescription). When I told Dr Bernes about these stocks, he immediately suggested I sell them off – I realized a $4,000 profit. I was lucky to have listened to Dr Bernes when I did, because I would have lost money had I held on to the stocks much longer. Dr Bernes suggested that I look into investing in the S&P 500 index fund, which is a collection of the 500 best companies in the United States. By investing in the S&P 500 index fund consistently, regardless of its price (which is called dollar-cost averaging), I could make a significant amount of money in the long term. Dr Bernes explained that it is not a very exciting way to invest, but it is the tried-and-true method of many wealthy people.

Ultimately, my discussion with Dr Bernes on finances was an incredibly important one. I was feeling down about my financial state during my depression, but with Dr Bernes' plan I was able to feel confident about the financial future I was working toward, and he gave me a lot to work on and build on. With the conclusion of mastering this area of The Octagon of Life, I was nearly fully recovered, but there was one more area I needed help with.

8. Mental Health Balance

Mental health balance was the last area of The Octagon of Life that Dr Bernes and I discussed. Because I am bipolar, I have a chemical imbalance in my brain that, if not treated, will cause mania or depression. For me, mental health balance meant taking regular medication. However, finding the right mixture of medication was a challenge. It would take over a year and 22 medication changes and adjustments before my prescription was right for me.

However, Dr Bernes explained that mental health balance was more than just taking medication. He reinforced that medication is an effective approach to getting a bipolar person out of mania or depression and back to a baseline or average lifestyle. But the whole point of The Octagon of Life was to take my life out of the average and into what Dr Bernes calls "the good life". For this area of The Octagon of Life, medication is foremost, but managing stress and practising self-care is important too.

At first, I used vaping as a self-care tactic to manage stress and to replace smoking marijuana. However, once I admitted to Dr Bernes that this was my strategy he had me quit vaping immediately. We both reached the conclusion that vaping serves no benefit, and that there are much healthier and safer self-care alternatives. He told me that we don't need to wait 50 years to determine that vaping is harmful for one's health.

To quit vaping, Dr Bernes suggested that I purchase some adult rehabilitation putty to keep my hands occupied when I felt stressed, and to practise mediation through diaphragmatic breathing. The combination of the putty and the breathing is a much healthier alternative to vaping and relieves more stress for me than vaping ever did.

Dr Bernes also told me that self-care included whatever I felt was a pleasurable, healthy activity. For me, this is playing softball, watching sports and listening to records. Self-care is important, because if my mental health balance is not the best it possibly can be, then everything in my life – from my relationships to my career – could suffer.

In addition, Dr Bernes said there is no shame in taking medication for a mental illness. He likened taking medication for the mental illness to taking insulin for diabetes. The diabetic has an imbalance in their body, while the bipolar person has an imbalance in their brain. The two conditions should be considered and respected equally. By this point in my recovery, I had long overcome the stigma of mental illness, but it was an important reminder, nonetheless.

Overall, with The Octagon of Life strategy, I was lifted out of depression into something known as "post-traumatic growth".

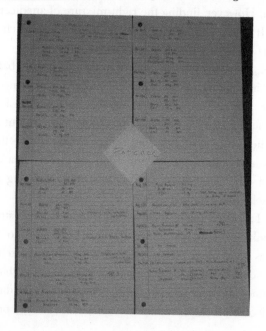

30

POST-TRAUMATIC GROWTH

Following The Octagon of Life plan, I began taking my life back. It was around summer 2018, and after my first semester back at school, that things started to come together again. I was taking two classes, and one was an English class that I thoroughly enjoyed. It was the first English class I had taken since changing my major back to English, and I knew right away that I had made the right decision. There was over a thousand pages of reading for the six-week course, but I excelled in it and got an A-, which I was thrilled with. I also took a class in Music Therapy, in which I achieved an A+. The following fall, I had another excellent semester, taking three classes and getting two A-s and one A.

When I visited Dr Palmer, he remarked at my success, saying, "Jason, you don't look like someone who has a mental illness." I was thrilled with this comment, and felt like I had gotten my life back.

Dr Bernes was also thrilled with my progress, my success at school and everything else in my life. He cited my accomplishments in one of our sessions, and said that what I was experiencing now was called "post-traumatic growth". Post-traumatic growth, he explained, occurs when a patient suffering from trauma, such as a manic episode, begins to experience a better life than prior to their diagnosis. He said this description fit me perfectly, as I was now excelling in virtually all areas of my life.

In January 2019, Dr Bernes asked me give a 45-minute presentation on my mental health journey and The Octagon of Life plan to his masters class of psychology students. It was my first real presentation in a long time, but I was more excited than nervous to share my story. The presentation went off without a hitch, and the class was amazed at my story – how I had gone from absolutely manic, to now getting good grades and living a healthy, balanced life. One woman in the audience came up to me afterwards and said, based on my presentation, I should write a book, as my story is one that needs to be told. And that is where this project began.

Manic Man: The Ultimate Exposure Therapy

I came to Dr Bernes with the idea of this book in February 2019. I told him that it was a ten-year goal of mine to write a book about my mental health journey. He thought this was a terrific idea, but said I wouldn't need ten years to complete it – I would need only six months. In late August 2019, I reached my goal of completing this project within six months. The project was emotionally tough at times, but overall, it has been the ultimate exposure therapy – I had to dive deeply into my manic episode and make sense of everything.

Writing this book also gave me the opportunity to mend some relationships, and help others come to terms with my behaviours during my manic episode. The book serves as a reminder to what I have been through, and how I never want to go back to the hospital ever again. I am proud that I have been able to put my thoughts to paper, and hope this book will be useful to those struggling with a mental illness. I hope it shows that things can get better, and that there is no ceiling on one's potential.

Final Word

Life can get better, whether you live with a mental illness or not – but it takes patience, commitment and some discipline. My advice for those newly diagnosed with a mental illness is to follow the plan laid out by your doctors; develop a care plan and a lifestyle that works for you, and then stick to it. Recovery from any significant mental health episode takes time, but things do come around, and life can get better even if you, too, are a Manic Man.

ACKNOWLEDGEMENTS

I would like to first thank my parents Leanna and Doug for their unconditional love for me. My manic episode was hard on them, as was the depression. They continued to show love and support throughout, thank you. The same goes for my sister Katherine and both sets of my grandparents: Dale Leffingwell, Beth Leffingwell, Joe Wegner and Shirley Wegner, thank you. It was the love I felt from my family that helped me in my darkest moments. Next, I would like to thank Dr. Kerry Bernes for pushing me to complete this project. When I came into his office with the idea of writing a book in the next ten years, his ambitious timeline of six months pushed me to complete the book in a timely manner. His help throughout was much appreciated. Thank you to my psychiatrist and his colleagues, who, through their tireless efforts, helped get me regulated and, after months of trying, finally got my medication right. Thank you to Trevor Hardy for being my mentor and to Greg Wolcott for inspiring me to become a teacher. Thank you, Mark Blankenstyn, Kevin McBeath and Jared Heidinger, for being there for me as your former student during my wild, manic episode. Thank you, Michael Clifford, for guiding me and being a friend when I exited the hospital. Thank you, Ross Delauw, Chase Bell and all the other friends who answered my many manic calls while I was in the hospital and for still being my friends after the fact. Thank you to my aunt Dianne Mensink for always thinking of me and supporting me through my depression. Thank you, Sydney Cleland, for featuring me in your Seeing Mental Illness project. The project was the first opportunity I took to speak out about my mental illness, thank you. Thank you, Bariyaa Ipaa, for taking the photographs provided in the book. Thank you to the rest of my family and friends who I have not mentioned. The love and support I have felt from family and friends throughout this entire process is humbling.

Thank you to Kayleigh McGowan, Jess Owen and the entire Cherish Editions team for believing in bringing my story to the public. You have all made the publishing process incredibly smooth, thank you.

Lastly, thank you, the reader, for reading my story. I hope you now realize that you can live a successful life regardless of any mental illness diagnosis.

ABOUT THE AUTHOR

Dr. Kerry Bernes

Dr. Kerry Bernes is a Board Certified Clinical Psychologist and Professor at the University of Lethbridge. He lives in Lethbridge, Alberta, Canada.

Jason Wegner

Jason Wegner is a student-teacher at the University of Lethbridge, an experienced public speaker and a first-time author. He was diagnosed with a severe mental illness, bipolar I disorder, in 2017 and, after recovering from his illness, began sharing his story of hope.

ABOUT CHERISH EDITIONS

Cherish Editions is a bespoke self-publishing service for authors of mental health, wellbeing and inspirational books.

As a division of Trigger Publishing, the UK's leading independent mental health and wellbeing publisher, we are experienced in creating and selling positive, responsible, important and inspirational books, which work to de-stigmatize the issues around mental health and improve the mental health and wellbeing of those who read our titles.

Founded by Adam Shaw, a mental health advocate, author and philanthropist, and leading psychologist Lauren Callaghan, Cherish Editions aims to publish books that provide advice, support and inspiration. We nurture our authors so that their stories can unfurl on the page, helping them to share their uplifting and moving stories.

Cherish Editions is unique in that a percentage of the profits from the sale of our books goes directly to leading mental health charity Shawmind, to deliver its vision to provide support for those experiencing mental ill health.

Find out more about Cherish Editions by visiting cherisheditions.com or by joining us on:
Twitter @cherisheditions
Facebook @cherisheditions
Instagram @cherisheditions

Cherish
EDITIONS

ABOUT SHAWMIND

A proportion of profits from the sale of all Trigger books go to their sister charity, Shawmind, also founded by Adam Shaw and Lauren Callaghan. The charity aims to ensure that everyone has access to mental health resources whenever they need them.

You can find out more about the work Shawmind do by visiting their website shawmind.org or joining them on:

Twitter @Shaw_Mind
Facebook @ShawmindUK
Instagram @Shaw_Mind

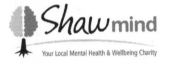

Lightning Source UK Ltd.
Milton Keynes UK
UKHW041257071021
391790UK00001B/169